Praise for *Spastic Quadriplegia—Bilateral Cerebral Palsy*

"Spastic Quadriplegia—Bilateral Cerebral Palsy is a comprehensive guide designed for families, health care professionals, and individuals living with this condition. It provides a holistic approach to the medical, developmental, and emotional aspects of spastic quadriplegia. The book offers insights into cerebral palsy's causes, symptoms, and treatments, emphasizing early diagnosis, intervention, and long-term management strategies. Personal stories are interwoven throughout the text, giving a human touch to the clinical information. The experience and expertise of the team at Gillette are evident in the excellent research and writing as well as in the structure, people-centered language, and compassion in each section."

HANK CHAMBERS, Professor of Clinical Orthopedic Surgery, University of California, San Diego; Medical Director of the Southern Family Center for Cerebral Palsy at Rady Children's Hospital, San Diego; Past President, American Academy of Cerebral Palsy and Developmental Medicine; Parent of adult son with CP, US

"Repeatedly in my reading of Spastic Quadriplegia, *I found myself wishing this book had been available 25 years ago. Parents facing a new diagnosis—or even parents who have walked this road for many years—will find the information easy to read and understand. Knowledge offers the power to prepare and to make educated decisions. Through this book, the team at Gillette Children's make that knowledge accessible to all, and thereby are certain to improve the lives of many."*

CAROL SHRADER, Mother of four, two with cerebral palsy; Policy Director for Delaware State Council for Persons with Disabilities; Freelance Writer and Speaker, US

"This book is a compelling must-read for families and nursing and medical professionals alike. It masterfully holds the space between the immense challenges of living with spastic quadriplegia and the everyday aspects of life—such as sleep, pain management, and digestion—that many take for granted but are essential to quality of life. The author reminds us to prioritize these often-overlooked needs while celebrating the joy, humour, and unique contributions that individuals with spastic quadriplegic cerebral palsy bring to the world."

IONA NOVAK, Cerebral Palsy Alliance Chair of Allied Health, The University of Sydney, Australia

T0325506

"This book opens with the observation that the parent is the expert of their child while the professional is the expert of the condition. In fact, the book will go a long way to help the parent—or, indeed, the adult with spastic quadriplegia—to become an expert in the condition themselves. It will equip parents and adults with the condition to understand the bigger picture of spastic quadriplegia, whether that's by using it to come to terms with the diagnosis and preparing for a lifetime of challenges ahead, or to dip back into after being bamboozled with potential risks, therapeutic recommendations, and alternative treatment options at a medical appointment. The book methodically breaks down the latest evidence-based research into laypersons' language. It is a must-have resource for every family of a person with spastic quadriplegia."

JOHN COUGHLAN, Secretary General, International Cerebral Palsy Society; Father of a young adult with spastic quadriplegia, Luxembourg

"Spastic Quadriplegia is a powerful and essential resource for anyone seeking to understand the complexities of this condition. With precision and compassion, it seamlessly blends cutting-edge research and clinical expertise with powerful personal narratives, creating a deeply impactful and accessible guide. What truly sets this book apart is its holistic perspective—it not only addresses the intricate medical and therapeutic challenges but also profoundly captures the strength and resilience of those living with spastic quadriplegia. This book is more than informative; it's transformative."

RACHEL BYRNE, Executive Director, Cerebral Palsy Foundation, US

"This book presents clear and concise explanations and eliminates the confusion caused by misinformation online. It has helped me realize that we are not alone; there are other families just like ours experiencing the same highs and lows, joys and sorrows. It will provide comfort and hope to families striving to adjust to a new and oftentimes difficult diagnosis."

KRISTEN STIER, Mother of a young adult with spastic quadriplegia, US

"I highly recommend this book for parents, clinicians, and individuals affected by spastic quadriplegia. The authors provide a clear explanation of the diagnosis and treatments, empowering parents to engage in meaningful discussions with medical professionals. The journeys of individuals and families are woven throughout the text, highlighting both their struggles and their joys. This book is a must-read!"

EILEEN FOWLER, Director, Research and Education, Center for Cerebral Palsy at UCLA/ Orthopaedic Institute for Children; Past President, American Academy of Cerebral Palsy and Developmental Medicine, US

"This comprehensive guide goes beyond the clinical picture of possibilities, issues, and conditions associated with a diagnosis of spastic quadriplegia. Cowritten by a parent and with personal stories from individuals and their families with this more complex form of cerebral palsy, it offers insider insight, practical tools, and helpful advice. This book is easy to navigate and covers the lifespan; it will serve as a great starting point when new issues arise and will guide the reader to the next step in care. This insight is backed up by facts and statistics that remind us that we are not alone on this journey."

JENNIFER LYNAM, Recreational Therapist; Parent of young adult with cerebral palsy, US

"I began to read this wonderful book whilst on a flight and was happily appreciating its content and layout when I came to one of the 'orange boxes': Kate's story describing Levi's birth and perinatal trauma and the impact on both her own and her husband's life. It suddenly hit me that Kate's story was also mine. Twenty-seven years ago, I, too, had a silent placental abruption during mid–first stage of labour with my beautiful son Conor. He was born covered in blood and clots and was unresponsive. Reading the book, I relived the sadness and pain and feelings of regret that 'it' had ever happened. But I am not stuck in that time. I have moved on hugely, have survived, and have ultimately accepted Conor for the person he is today. Indeed, I very rarely think of what could/should have been. He lives in supported accommodation and is hugely loved by his dedicated carers. He is also very much loved and a vital part of our family. He visits on Sundays, and we go for walks; he tastes small amounts of chocolate, and he even goes to the pub with us while we have a drink!

"The family story told throughout the book contains wisdom and honest insights into the feelings and thoughts that accompany parents on this journey with a disabled child; they are invaluable for families and clinicians alike. It addresses what to consider when making the many care decisions, such as whether there is benefit in continuing a specific therapy if the child is not enjoying it. The photos brought the family story to life and reminded me of the many hours I spent swimming with Conor during his baby days. He loved the warmth of the water and the freedom that the buoyancy gave him.

"The book is beautifully laid out and so user-friendly; it's suitable for all levels of knowledge, and you can dip into whichever part of the book that answers your current query, whether it is in relation to feeding, growth, respiratory issues, mobility, surgery, or more. The photographs are really wonderful with so many smiling faces using the many assistive/adaptive technologies available today.

"The section on transition to adulthood raises a very important issue and is an area every country needs to work on. It is so important that parents be allowed to enjoy their late-middle and old age without having to worry about how their child will be looked after when they are no longer able to.

"Congratulations on a really wonderful book!"

DR. ÍDE NICDHONNCHA HICKEY, Principal Medical Officer, Sligo; Mother of son with spastic quadriplegia, Ireland

SPASTIC QUADRIPLEGIA BILATERAL CEREBRAL PALSY

SPASTIC QUADRIPLEGIA

Bilateral Cerebral Palsy

Understanding and
managing the condition
across the lifespan:
A practical guide for families

Marcie Ward, MD
Lily Collison, MA, MSc
Cheryl Tveit, RN, MSN, CNML
Kate Edin, Parent

Edited by
Elizabeth R. Boyer, PhD
Tom F. Novacheck, MD
GILLETTE CHILDREN'S

Gillette Children's Healthcare Press
200 University Avenue East
St Paul, MN 55101
www.GilletteChildrensHealthcarePress.org
HealthcarePress@gillettechildrens.com

ISBN 978-1-952181-17-7 (paperback)
ISBN 978-1-952181-18-4 (e-book)
LIBRARY OF CONGRESS CONTROL NUMBER 2024941674

COPYEDITING BY Ruth Wilson
ORIGINAL ILLUSTRATIONS BY Olwyn Roche
COVER AND INTERIOR DESIGN BY Jazmin Welch
PROOFREADING BY Ruth Wilson
INDEX BY Audrey McClellan

Printed by Hobbs the Printers Ltd, Totton, Hampshire, UK

For information about distribution or special discounts for bulk purchases, please contact:
Mac Keith Press
2nd Floor, Rankin Building
139-143 Bermondsey Street
London, SE1 3UW
www.mackeith.co.uk
admin@mackeith.co.uk

The views and opinions expressed herein are those of the authors and Gillette Children's Healthcare Press and do not necessarily represent those of Mac Keith Press.

To individuals and families whose lives are affected by these conditions, to professionals who serve our community, and to all clinicians and researchers who push the knowledge base forward, we hope the books in this Healthcare Series serve you very well.

Gillette Children's acknowledges a grant from the Cerebral Palsy Foundation for the writing of this book.

All proceeds from the books in this series at Gillette Children's go to research.

All information contained in this book is for educational purposes only. For specific medical advice and treatment, please consult a qualified health care professional. The information in this book is not intended as a substitute for consultation with your health care professional.

Contents

APPENDICES (ONLINE)

Appendix 1: Measurement tools
Appendix 2: Bones, joints, muscles, and movements
Appendix 3: Epilepsy management
Appendix 4: Scoliosis management

Authors and Editors

Marcie Ward, MD, Pediatric Rehabilitation Medicine Physician, Gillette Children's

Lily Collison, MA, MSc, Program Director, Gillette Children's Healthcare Press

Cheryl Tveit, RN, MSN, CNML, Principal Writer, Gillette Children's Healthcare Press

Kate Edin, Parent

Elizabeth R. Boyer, PhD, Clinical Scientist, Gillette Children's

Tom F. Novacheck, MD, Medical Director of Integrated Care Services, Gillette Children's; Professor of Orthopedics, University of Minnesota; and Past President, American Academy for Cerebral Palsy and Developmental Medicine

Series Foreword

You hold in your hands one book in the Gillette Children's Healthcare Series. This series was inspired by multiple factors.

It started with Lily Collison writing the first book in the series, *Spastic Diplegia–Bilateral Cerebral Palsy*. Lily has a background in medical science and is the parent of a now adult son who has spastic diplegia. Lily was convincing at the time about the value of such a book, and with the publication of that book in 2020, Gillette Children's became one of the first children's hospitals in the world to set up its own publishing arm—Gillette Children's Healthcare Press. *Spastic Diplegia–Bilateral Cerebral Palsy* received very positive reviews from both families and professionals and achieved strong sales. Unsolicited requests came in from diverse organizations across the globe for translation rights, and feedback from families told us there was a demand for books relevant to other conditions.

We listened.

We were convinced of the value of expanding from one book into a series to reflect Gillette Children's strong commitment to worldwide education. In 2021, Lily joined the press as Program Director, and very quickly, Gillette Children's formed teams to write the Healthcare Series. The series includes, in order of publication:

- *Craniosynostosis*
- *Idiopathic Scoliosis*
- *Spastic Hemiplegia—Unilateral Cerebral Palsy*
- *Spastic Quadriplegia—Bilateral Cerebral Palsy*
- *Spastic Diplegia—Bilateral Cerebral Palsy, second edition*
- *Epilepsy*
- *Spina Bifida*
- *Osteogenesis Imperfecta*
- *Scoliosis—Congenital, Neuromuscular, Syndromic, and Other Causes*

The books address each condition detailing both the medical and human story.

Mac Keith Press, long-time publisher of books on disability and the journal *Developmental Medicine and Child Neurology*, is co-publishing this series with Gillette Children's Healthcare Press.

Families and professionals working well together is key to best management of any condition. The parent is the expert of their child while the professional is the expert of the condition. These books underscore the importance of that family and professional partnership. For each title in the series, medical professionals at Gillette Children's have led the writing, and families contributed the lived experience.

These books have been written in the United States with an international lens and citing international research. However, there isn't always strong evidence to create consensus in medicine, so others may take a different view.

We hope you find the book you hold in your hands to be of great value. We collectively strive to optimize outcomes for children, adolescents, and adults living with these childhood-acquired and largely lifelong conditions.

Dr. Tom F. Novacheck

Series Introduction

The Healthcare Series seeks to optimize outcomes for those who live with childhood-acquired physical and/or neurological conditions. The conditions addressed in this series of books are complex and often have many associated challenges. Although the books focus on the biomedical aspects of each condition, we endeavor to address each condition as holistically as possible. Since the majority of people with these conditions have them for life, the life course is addressed including transition and aging issues.

Who are these books for?

These books are written for an international audience. They are primarily written for parents of young children, but also for adolescents and adults who have the condition. They are written for members of multidisciplinary teams and researchers. Finally, they are written for others, including extended family members, teachers, and students taking courses in the fields of medicine, allied health care, and education.

A worldview

The books in the series focus on evidence-based best practice, which we acknowledge is not available everywhere. It is mostly available in high-income countries (at least in urban areas, though even there, not always), but many families live away from centers of good care.

We also acknowledge that the majority of people with disabilities live in low- and middle-income countries. Improving the lives of all those with disabilities across the globe is an important goal. Developing scalable, affordable interventions is a crucial step toward achieving this. Nonetheless, the best interventions will fail if we do not first address the social determinants of health—the economic, social, and environmental conditions in which people live that shape their overall health and well-being.

No family reading these books should ever feel they have failed their child. We all struggle to do our best for our children within the limitations of our various resources and situations. Indeed, the advocacy role these books may play may help families and professionals lobby in unison for best care.

International Classification of Functioning, Disability and Health

The writing of the series of books has been informed by the International Classification of Functioning, Disability and Health (ICF).[1] The framework explains the impact of a health condition at different levels and how those levels are interconnected. It tells us to look at the full picture—to look at the person with a disability in their life situation.

The framework shows that every human being can experience a decrease in health and thereby experience some disability. It is not something that happens only to a minority of people. The ICF thus "mainstreams" disability and recognizes it as a widespread human experience.

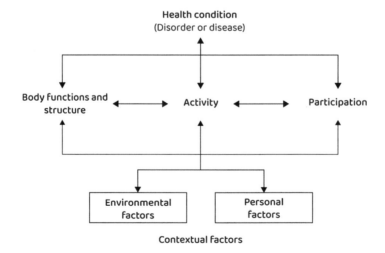

International Classification of Functioning, Disability and Health (ICF). Reproduced with kind permission from WHO.

In health care, there has been a shift away from focusing almost exclusively on correcting issues that cause the individual's functional problems to focusing also on the individual's activity and participation. These books embrace maximizing participation for all people living with disability.

The family

For simplicity, throughout the series we refer to "parents" and "children"; we acknowledge, however, that family structures vary. "Parent" is used as a generic term that includes grandparents, relatives, and carers (caregivers) who are raising a child. Throughout the series, we refer to male and female as the biologic sex assigned at birth. We acknowledge that this does not equate to gender identity or sexual orientation, and we respect the individuality of each person. Throughout the series we have included both "person with disability" and "disabled person," recognizing that both terms are used.

Caring for a child with a disability can be challenging and overwhelming. Having a strong social support system in place can make a difference. For the parent, balancing the needs of the child with a disability with the needs of siblings—while also meeting employment demands, nurturing a relationship with a significant other, and caring for aging parents—can sometimes feel like an enormous juggling act. Siblings may feel neglected or overlooked because of the increased attention given to the disabled child. It is crucial for parents to allocate time and resources to ensure that siblings feel valued and included in the family dynamics. Engaging siblings in the care and support of the disabled child can help foster a sense of unity and empathy within the family.

A particular challenge for a child and adolescent who has a disability, and their parent, is balancing school attendance (for both academic and social purposes) with clinical appointments and surgery. Appointments outside of school hours are encouraged. School is important because the cognitive and social abilities developed there help maximize employment opportunities when employment is a realistic goal. Indeed, technology has eliminated barriers and created opportunities that did not exist even 10 years ago.

Parents also need to find a way to prioritize self-care. Neglecting their own well-being can have detrimental effects on their mental and physical health. Think of the safety advice on an airplane: you are told that you must put on your own oxygen mask before putting on your child's. It's the same when caring for a child with a disability; parents need to take care of themselves in order to effectively care for their child *and* family. Friends, support groups, or mental health professionals can provide an outlet for parents to express their emotions, gain valuable insights, and find solace in knowing that they are not alone in their journey.

For those of you reading this book who have the condition, we hope this book gives you insights into its many nuances and complexities, acknowledges you as an expert in your own care, and provides a road map and framework for you to advocate for your needs.

Last words

This series of books seeks to be an invaluable educational resource. All proceeds from the series at Gillette Children's go to research.

Chapter 1

Cerebral palsy

Introduction

So be sure when you step.
Step with care and great tact
and remember that Life's
a Great Balancing Act …
And will you succeed?
Yes! You will, indeed!
(98 and ¾ percent guaranteed.)
Kid, you'll move mountains!
Dr. Seuss

To fully understand spastic quadriplegia, it is worth first having an understanding of the umbrella term "cerebral palsy" (CP). "Cerebral" refers to a specific part of the brain (the cerebrum) and "palsy" literally means paralysis (cerebrum paralysis). Although paralysis describes something different from the typical features of CP, it is the origin of the term "palsy."

CP was first described in 1861 by an English doctor, William Little, and for many years it was known as "Little's disease." Over the years there has been much discussion of the definition of CP, and different definitions have been adopted and later discarded. Following is the most recently adopted definition, published in 2007:

> *Cerebral palsy describes a group of permanent disorders of the development of movement and posture, causing activity limitation, that are attributed to non-progressive disturbances that occurred in the developing fetal or infant brain. The motor disorders of cerebral palsy are often accompanied by disturbances of sensation, perception, cognition, communication, behaviour, by epilepsy and by secondary musculoskeletal problems.*[2]

In other words, CP is a *group* of conditions caused by an injury to the developing brain, which can result in a variety of motor and other problems that affect how the child functions. Because the injury occurs in a *developing brain and growing child*, problems often change over time, even though the brain injury itself is unchanging. Table 1.1.1 explains the terms used in the definition of CP above, in order.

Table 1.1.1 Explanation of terms in definition of CP

TERMS	EXPLANATION
Cerebral	"Cerebral" refers to the cerebrum, one of the major areas of the brain responsible for the control of movement.
Palsy	"Palsy" means paralysis, that is, an inability to activate muscles by the nervous system, though paralysis by pure definition is not a feature of CP.
Group	CP is not a single condition, unlike conditions such as type 1 diabetes. Rather, CP is a group of conditions. The location, timing, and type of brain injury vary, as do the resulting effects.
Permanent	The brain injury remains for life; CP is a permanent, lifelong condition.
Disorders	A disorder is a disruption in the usual orderly process. To meet the definition of CP, the disorder must cause activity limitation.
Posture	Posture is the way a person holds their body when, for example, standing, sitting, or moving.

Cont'd.

TERMS	EXPLANATION
Activity limitation	An activity is the execution of a task or action by an individual. Activity limitations are difficulties an individual may have in doing activities. Walking with difficulty is an example.
Nonprogressive	The brain injury does not worsen, but its effects can develop or evolve over time.
Developing fetal or infant brain	The brain of a fetus or infant has not finished developing all its neural connections and is therefore immature. An injury to an immature brain is different from an injury to a mature brain.
Motor disorders	Motor disorders are conditions affecting the ability to move and the quality of those movements.
Sensation	"Sensation" can be defined as a physical feeling or perception arising from something that happens to or that comes in contact with the body.
Perception	Perception is the ability to incorporate and interpret sensory and/or cognitive information.
Cognition	"Cognition" means the mental action or process of acquiring knowledge and understanding through thought, experience, and the senses.
Communication	Communication is the imparting or exchanging of information.
Behavior	"Behavior" refers to the way a person acts or conducts themselves.
Epilepsy	Epilepsy is a neurological disorder in which brain electrical activity becomes abnormal, causing seizures or periods of unusual behavior, sensations, and sometimes loss of awareness.
Secondary musculoskeletal problems	"Musculoskeletal" refers to both the muscles and the skeleton (i.e., the muscles, bones, joints, and their related structures). Musculoskeletal problems appear with time and growth and are therefore termed "secondary problems." They develop as a consequence of the brain injury. People with CP may develop a variety of musculoskeletal problems, such as bone torsion (twist), or muscle contracture (a limitation of range of motion of a joint).

Adapted from Rosenbaum and colleagues.[2]

CP is the most common cause of physical disability in children.[3] It is acquired during pregnancy, birth, or in early childhood, and it is a lifelong condition. There is currently no cure, nor is one imminent, but good management and treatment can help alleviate some or many of the effects of the brain injury.

When the brain injury occurs is important. The consequences of a brain injury to a fetus developing in the uterus are generally different from those of a brain injury sustained at birth, which in turn are different from those of a brain injury acquired during infancy. The European and Australian Cerebral Palsy Registers use two years of age as the cutoff for applying the diagnosis of CP.[4,5] A brain injury occurring after two years of age is called an "acquired brain injury." This two-year cutoff is applied because of the differences in brain maturity relative to when the brain injury occurs.

Although the development of movement and posture is affected in individuals with CP, as seen above, other body systems can also be affected.

How to read this book

To help you navigate the information in this book, it has been organized so that you can read it from beginning to end or, alternatively, dip into different sections and chapters independently. Because much of the information builds on previous sections and chapters, it is best to first read the book in its entirety to get an overall sense of the condition. After that, you can return to the parts that are relevant to you, knowing that you can ignore other sections or revisit them if and when they do become relevant.

This chapter addresses the overall condition of CP. Chapter 2 addresses spastic quadriplegia. Chapters 3 to 6 address the overall management of spastic quadriplegia. Chapter 7 addresses alternative and complementary treatments. Chapter 8 addresses transition to adulthood, and adulthood for individuals with spastic quadriplegia is addressed in Chapter 9.

Throughout Chapters 1 to 9, medical information is interspersed with personal lived experience. Orange boxes are used to highlight the personal story. Chapter 10 is devoted to vignettes from individuals and families around the globe. Chapter 11 provides further reading and research.

At the back of the book, you'll find a glossary of key terms.

A companion website for this book is available at www.Gillette ChildrensHealthcarePress.org. This website contains some useful web resources and appendices. A QR code to access **Useful web resources** is included below.

It may be helpful to discuss any questions you may have from reading this book with your medical professional.

Final words

Before delving in, it is worth highlighting the following points, presented in no particular order:

- You may feel a mixture of feelings, some positive, some negative, and even conflicting feelings at the same time. That's okay. Sometimes you may be coping very well, other times not. That's okay too. Try to get as much support as you can. Never forget to first take care of yourself.
- You may feel incredibly overwhelmed by the sheer number of issues a diagnosis of spastic quadriplegia brings, and it can be very hard to prioritize what to tackle first, what can wait, and how to navigate everything all at once. You may feel overwhelmed that a diagnosis of spastic quadriplegia likely brings a lifetime of care; that there's a lot to organize including finding good people to help, sorting through finance and insurance issues, navigating respite, multiple appointments, and more. *We understand you and we are here to help you navigate this.*
- Early intervention is important. For example, early access to assistive technology for mobility, for communication, and for vision helps to maximize the child's ability to interact, to participate, and to learn.
- Inclusion in education early and throughout all school years is important. No child or adolescent with spastic quadriplegia should

be isolated. This will require a team approach and trialing different options to see what works best.

- Spend time exploring things that you or your child loves. Don't let therapy become the main focus or an end in itself. Many families spend so much time with therapies they don't take time to have fun and do the things they enjoy.
- There are probably far more adaptive recreational activities available to individuals with spastic quadriplegia than you think. See Chapter 4.
- Hanging out with friends and family, slowing down, and simply ensuring the individual with spastic quadriplegia is included is very important.
- Independence is a topic that you may hear a lot about, but interdependence may, in fact, be the key. In life, all of us are interdependent to varying degrees; no one is an island.
- Spastic quadriplegia is a complex condition. It is hoped that with more research, understanding will increase, and more interventions will become available. While being realistic, set your expectations high to get the best for you or your loved one with spastic quadriplegia.

USEFUL WEB RESOURCES

Levi and his identical twin brother, Cam, were born at 27 weeks gestation. Back in my 20s, I had some precancerous cells removed from my cervix through a procedure known as a cold-knife conization. Unbeknownst to me, that included removing my entire external cervix. I was lucky enough to have found out about my compromised cervix during a fertility examination prior to becoming pregnant. My OB-GYN foresaw that the removal of my cervix would make it quite difficult to carry a child to term and suggested I think about getting a cerclage (a procedure to sew up the cervix to prevent premature delivery) after I got pregnant.

In doing some research, I learned about a prepregnancy cerclage called a TAC. In this procedure, the transabdominal cerclage would be placed around the upper cervix and would perform the job of holding in a baby should I become pregnant. I flew to Chicago to have a world-renowned doctor place my TAC, and I subsequently used IUI (intrauterine insemination) to become pregnant, as my OB-GYN wanted to control as much of my pregnancy as possible.

During the cycle I got pregnant with Levi, there was only one egg follicle "ripe" enough for fertilization, so everyone was very surprised at my first ultrasound when we saw two gestational sacs! From that moment, my pregnancy went from complicated to high risk, and I switched from being attended by my regular OB-GYN to a maternal fetal medicine center. I had an irritable uterus and contracted frequently from about 14 weeks until delivery. I was on bed rest from about 20 weeks on.

At my ultrasound at week 26, my doctor released me from bed rest, but she told me to stay low-key and not play any sports. Three days later, my water broke, and in that moment the entire trajectory of my life was rerouted.

Twin A, Cameron, was the one whose water had broken. Levi was still safe and sound in his comfy bag of water. Because I had the TAC, doctors knew I would not be able to deliver naturally and would require an emergency C-section before either the babies or I got an infection. I was given a brief explanation of the neonatal intensive care unit (NICU) and handed more printouts and pamphlets about prematurity than I knew what to do with. Scared about the future, but knowing I was in the right hospital, I delivered around 9 a.m. on July 19, 2009. Cam and

Levi were both born within minutes of each other, Cam weighing 2 lb 5 oz, and Levi slightly smaller at 2 lb 2oz.

All was well for the first few hours, but then the boys began to struggle to breathe, so they both had breathing tubes inserted. In the following days, the babies did well, their brain scans were clear, and everything looked great. I began to think that everything would be okay; we would stay in the NICU until the boys were bigger, and then we would go home.

At two weeks old, Levi began to get sick. It happened quickly and was untraditional in presentation (being "untraditional" would become Levi's pattern for his entire life). His temperature spiked and his heart rate increased. He also wasn't tolerating his feeds. The doctors suspected necrotizing enterocolitis, or NEC, an infection that is prevalent in the NICU. They predicted his illness would follow the normal course and that they would have a few days to combat the illness with antibiotics.

But Levi didn't do what was expected, and within hours he was rushed into surgery because his bowels had perforated due to the NEC. The surgeon was able to remove all the dead intestine and brought the ends of his living intestine out to the surface through an ostomy (a surgically created opening). The surgery was tough, but brain scans still showed no hemorrhages or damage.

The next day, when Cam began to present with the same signs of fever and increased heart rate, doctors immediately suspected NEC and placed him on high-powered antibiotics and the JET vent (high-frequency air delivery). With that support, Cam's little body was able to fight off the infection.

What happened next is important to understanding how Levi wound up with CP. At about eight weeks old, he was ready to have his ostomy taken down[*] and the ends of his intestines reconnected. The surgery was supposed to be routine, but as with everything Levi experiences, it did not go as expected. The surgeon found more necrotic tissue that needed to be removed, and Levi's little body couldn't maintain his blood

---

[*] Surgery to remove or close a previously surgically created opening (ostomy) in the abdomen. Ostomy takedown surgery is to restore bowel function by reconnecting the intestines and eliminating the need for collection of stool in an external bag.

pressure during the extensive procedure. It was after this surgery that his brain scans looked different from his brother's, and we pinpoint that as when Levi's CP came into being.

When the doctors first discussed the brain scan with me, they threw around acronyms like CP and PVL (periventricular leukomalacia, or injury to the white matter in the brain) and reminded me that no one can predict how a child with a brain scan like Levi's would do. They said they thought he would likely have ankle and foot issues based on the imaging. The white matter in Levi's brain was impacted by the PVL, but the gray matter was not, which was significant when Levi was eventually diagnosed with CP.

I went home and researched cerebral palsy and PVL. I was overwhelmed and unsure of what to do. Although I did not know it at the time, Levi's birth was also a second birth for me. I had gone from being a typical 29-year-old first-time mom of twins to being a special needs mama bear whose life focus was now learning how to support, empower, and advocate for her child.

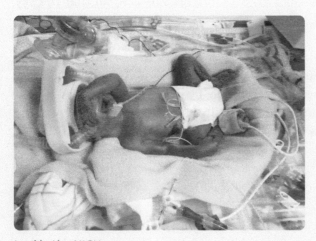

Levi in the NICU.

The nervous system

The Brain—is wider than the Sky
Emily Dickinson

CP results from an injury to the developing fetal or young child's brain, or a difference in how the fetal brain forms. A basic understanding of the nervous system is useful to help understand the effects of the brain injury. This section briefly explains the main components of the nervous system.

The nervous system is composed of the:

- Central nervous system (CNS)—the brain and spinal cord.
- Peripheral nervous system (PNS)—a large network of nerves that carry messages between the CNS and the rest of the body. The autonomic nervous system is part of the PNS; it controls involuntary functions of the brain and body, such as breathing, heart rate, and digestion.

See Figure 1.2.1.

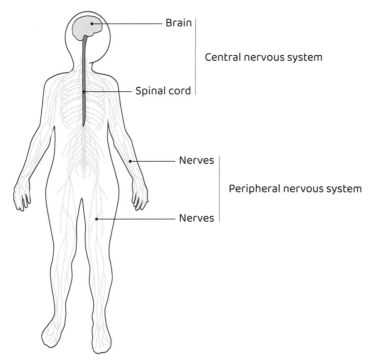

Figure 1.2.1 The nervous system.

Nerve cells

The nerve cell (also known as "neuron" or "neurone") is the basic unit of the nervous system. Nerve cells carry information between the CNS and the rest of the body as electrical impulses. There are three types of nerve cells:

- Motor nerve cells, which take information from the CNS to a muscle or gland
- Sensory nerve cells, which do the opposite, taking messages from the rest of the body to the CNS
- Interneurons (also known as "relay neurons"), which carry information between nerve cells

Figure 1.2.2 shows a typical nerve cell. Note the cell body and axon. Information enters the nerve cell through the dendrites and cell body, and exits via the axonal endings. The cell bodies form the gray matter of the brain, and the axons form the white matter, or the communication tracts.

The whitish color of the white matter is due to the fatty substance, called "myelin," that covers the axons; this insulates and speeds up the transmission of electrical impulses. Nerve cells receive, interpret, and transfer messages as electrical impulses. These electrical impulses form the brain's electrical activity, which can be measured and recorded on an electroencephalogram (EEG).

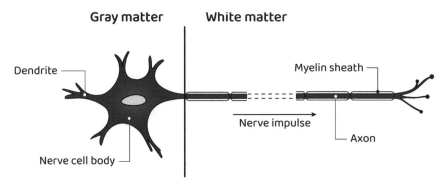

Figure 1.2.2 Nerve cell. Adapted with kind permission from *The Identification and Treatment of Gait Problems in Cerebral Palsy*, 2nd edition, edited by James Gage et al. (2009). Mac Keith Press.

Brain structure and functions

The brain is housed inside the cranium, a bony covering that protects the brain from external injury. Together, the cranium and the bones that protect the face make up the skull.

The brain is divided into several distinct parts that serve important functions. See Figure 1.2.3.

The *cerebrum* is the front and upper part of the brain. The cerebral cortex (the outer layer, the surface of the brain) is the gray matter where the cell bodies of the nerve cells are found. The cerebral cortex has a large surface area and, due to its folds, it appears wrinkled. Different regions of the cerebral cortex have different functions.

The *cerebellum* is located at the back of the brain, under the cerebrum, and helps with maintaining balance and posture, coordination, and fine motor movements.

The *brain stem* is the bottom part of the brain that connects the cerebrum to the *spinal cord*. It also serves as a relay station for messages between different parts of the body and the cerebral cortex. Many functions responsible for survival are located here (e.g., breathing and heart rate).

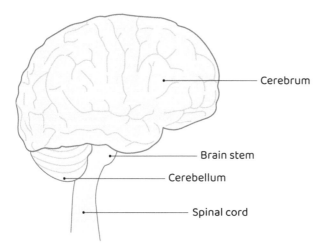

Cerebrum

Brain stem

Cerebellum

Spinal cord

Figure 1.2.3 Parts of the brain.

The cerebrum is divided in two halves, referred to as hemispheres (see Figure 1.2.4). In general, the right half controls the left side of the body, and the left half controls the right side of the body. Therefore, damage on the right side of the cerebrum will impact the left side of the body and vice versa. Communication between the two halves occurs in the corpus callosum, located in the center of the cerebrum.

The *basal ganglia* and *thalamus* are located in the middle of the cerebrum, deep beneath the cerebral cortex. The basal ganglia are important in the control of movement, including motor learning and planning. The thalamus is sometimes referred to as a relay station—it relays various sensory information (e.g., sight, sound, touch) to the cerebral cortex from the rest of the body.

Cerebrospinal fluid is found within the brain and around the spinal cord. It is produced within channels in the brain, called ventricles. Cerebrospinal fluid helps protect the brain and spinal cord from injury.

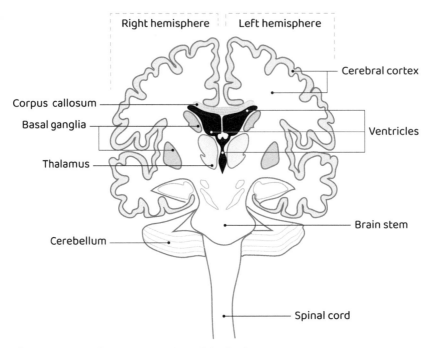

Figure 1.2.4 Vertical cross-section of the brain.

Causes, risk factors, and prevalence

The little reed, bending to the force of the wind, soon stood upright again when the storm had passed over.

Aesop

The US Centers for Disease Control and Prevention (CDC) defines "cause" as:

> *A factor (characteristic, behavior, event, etc.) that directly influences the occurrence of disease. A reduction of the factor in the population should lead to a reduction in the occurrence of disease.*

It defines "risk factor" as:

> *An aspect of personal behavior or lifestyle, an environmental exposure, or an inborn or inherited characteristic that is associated with an increased occurrence of disease or other health-related event or condition.*[6]

Causes thus have a stronger relationship with CP than do risk factors. A significant stroke in the infant's brain, for example, is a cause of CP.

Preterm birth (i.e., less than 37 weeks gestation) is a risk factor but not a cause of CP—in other words, not every preterm infant is found to have CP. There are many possible causes of brain injury, including events during fetal development, pregnancy, birth, or early infant life. Much is known about the causes and risk factors for CP, but more remains unknown.

Causes

Data from Australia shows that 94 percent of children with CP had a brain injury in the prenatal or perinatal periods (i.e., during pregnancy and up to the first 28 days after birth), while only 6 percent had a recognized postnatal brain injury (acquired more than 28 days after birth and before two years of age).[4] Seventy to 80 percent of CP cases are associated with prenatal factors, and birth asphyxia (lack of oxygen during birth) plays a relatively minor role.[7]

There are many causes of brain injury, including:

- **Hypoxia-ischemia:** from hypoxia, which is a deficiency of oxygen, and ischemia, which is reduced blood flow to the brain. Hypoxia-ischemia is a combination of both terms
- **Hemorrhage:** bleeding in the brain, also termed a "cerebral vascular accident" (CVA) or a stroke
- **Infection**
- **Abnormalities in brain development**[7]

A decrease in oxygen and insufficient blood supply to the brain have different effects in preterm infants compared with term infants due to the different stages of their brain development. As noted in section 1.2, the nerve cell bodies form the gray matter while axons form the white matter or the communication tracts. It has been found that white matter injuries predominate in infants born preterm, whereas gray matter injuries are more common in infants born at term.[7]

Approximately 90 percent of cases of CP result from healthy brain tissue becoming damaged rather than from abnormalities in brain development.[3] The cause of CP in an individual child is very often unknown.[8,9]

Risk factors

Infants who are born preterm (earlier than 37 weeks) or who have low birth weight have a higher risk of CP.[10] Twins and other multiple-birth siblings are at particular risk because they tend to be born early and at lower birth weights. Australian data shows that:[4]

- Forty-three percent of births of children with CP were preterm compared to 9 percent in the typical population.
- Forty-three percent of children with CP were born with low birth weight (under 2,500 grams, or 5.5 lb) compared to 7 percent in the typical population.
- The prevalence of children with CP was higher for twin than singleton births. This is why single embryo transfer in assisted reproductive technology (ART)* is strongly encouraged.[11,12]

In addition to the above, other risk factors for CP include the following (not an exhaustive list):[7]

- Prior to conception:
  - Young or advanced maternal age
  - A history of stillbirth or multiple miscarriages
  - Low socioeconomic status
  - Genetic factors
- During pregnancy:
  - Male sex: Males account for a greater proportion of individuals with CP than females. Australia data shows that 58 percent of those with CP were male.[4]
  - TORCH complex: TORCH is an acronym used to refer to a group of infections that can affect a developing fetus or a newborn: Toxoplasmosis (caused by a parasite), Other infections, Rubella (also known as German measles), Cytomegalovirus, and Herpes simplex virus.
  - Maternal thyroid disorder.
  - Pre-eclampsia (high blood pressure that can pose serious risks to both mother and fetus if left untreated).

---

* A broad term encompassing various fertility treatments, including in vitro fertilization, intrauterine insemination, and egg freezing.

      o   Placenta problems (e.g., placenta previa, placenta abruption).*
- Around the time of birth and during the neonatal (newborn) period:
  - o   An acute hypoxic event (lack of oxygen) during birth
  - o   Meconium aspiration†
  - o   Seizures
  - o   Low blood sugar

Some risk factors are declining, but others are increasing. Although any one risk factor may cause CP, if that factor is severe enough, it is more often caused by the combination of multiple risk factors.[13] Although preterm birth is a large risk factor for CP, it's the causal pathways that have led to it, or the consequences of it, that may cause the CP, rather than the preterm birth itself.

Mutations or changes in the genes involved in brain development or function (either inherited or *de novo,* which is a change in a gene that appears for the first time in a child but is not present in either parent) can increase susceptibility to CP. These genetic risk factors may affect the severity of symptoms, the specific type of CP, or the likelihood of associated conditions. Genetic risk factors may interact with other risk factors, highlighting the complex interplay between multiple risk factors in determining the development of the condition.

In low- and middle-income countries, causes and risk factors differ. In these countries, few preterm infants survive. Birth asphyxia is more common due to complications during labor or delivery. Also more common is Rhesus incompatibility (a mismatch in the Rhesus blood group system between the mother and the fetus). As well, a higher proportion of postnatally acquired CP is associated with infections such as meningitis, septicemia, and malaria.[7]

---

* "Placenta previa" means the placenta partially or fully covers the cervix. It can lead to bleeding and complications during birth. "Placenta abruption" means the placenta detaches from the uterus before the infant is born, with potentially life-threatening risks for both the mother and infant. It requires immediate medical attention.

† When a newborn breathes in a mixture of amniotic fluid (fluid that was surrounding the fetus in the uterus) and stool during or shortly after birth, potentially causing respiratory issues.

Prevalence

The prevalence of a condition is how many people in a defined population have the condition at a specific point in time. Prevalence can vary geographically and change over time because of medical advances and social and economic development.

Having an understanding of prevalence, along with causes and risk factors, can help with prevention of CP. A systematic review[*] of interventions for prevention and treatment of CP reported that effective prenatal interventions include corticosteroids and magnesium sulfate; effective neonatal (newborn) interventions include caffeine (methylxanthine) and hypothermia.[†14]

CP registers[‡] are essential for tracking and analyzing the prevalence and trends of CP in populations. They provide researchers and health care providers with critical data on the incidence, types, severity, and outcomes of CP, which can lead to improved health care policies and practices. It would be very helpful if, once a child is diagnosed with CP, parents would give consent to have their child added to a CP register.

Many countries maintain CP registers. There are two major networks of registers: the Surveillance of Cerebral Palsy in Europe (SCPE, established in 1998) and the Australian Cerebral Palsy Register (ACPR, established in 2007). A newer network of registers was established in 2018: the Global Low- and Middle-Income Countries CP Register (GLM CPR). There is no single national CP register in the US. There, instead, CP data is often collected and maintained by various state or regional programs, research facilities, or health care centers.

The current CP birth prevalence in high-income countries is declining and is now 1.6 per 1,000 live births (data 1995 to 2014).[5] However, in the US, prevalence was found to be higher at 2.9 per 1,000 eight-year-olds (2010 data)[15] and 3.2 per 1,000 3- to 17-year-olds (2009–2016 data).[16]

---

[*] A systematic review summarizes the results of a number of scientific studies.

[†] The controlled cooling of a newborn's body temperature.[20]

[‡] Confidential databases that store important data about individuals with CP.

Current CP birth prevalence is also higher in low- and middle-income countries.[5] The prevalence in rural Bangladesh was reported as 3.4 per 1,000 children, and the majority had potentially preventable risk factors.[17] For example, only 30 percent of mothers received regular prenatal care.[17]

The most recent report from the Australian Cerebral Palsy Register shows a decrease in both prevalence and severity of CP between 1997 and 2016.[4] The decrease in prevalence was from 2.4 to 1.5 per 1,000 live births, a decrease of almost 40 percent. The decrease in severity was evidenced by a decrease in the proportion of children with greater functional mobility challenges, and in the proportion of children with epilepsy or intellectual impairment. This is encouraging because it suggests that with the application of resources, prevalence and severity may be able to be reduced in other countries.

Unfortunately, funding for CP research is very low. Although the reported prevalence of CP is double that of Down syndrome,[18] funding awarded for CP research in 2023 ($30 million) was significantly lower than for Down syndrome research ($133 million).[19]

Diagnosis

Acceptance is knowing that grief is a raging river. And you have to
get into it. Because when you do, it carries you to the next place.
It eventually takes you to open land, somewhere where it will
turn out OK in the end.

Simone George

There is no single test to confirm CP, unlike other conditions such as
type 1 diabetes, which is confirmed through a simple blood test for
glucose, or Down syndrome, which is confirmed through a genetic test.
Recall that CP is not a single condition; rather, it is a group of conditions. The location, timing, and type of brain injury vary, and the
resulting effects of the brain injury are also varied.

Until recently, a diagnosis of CP was generally made between 12 and
24 months based on a combination of clinical signs (e.g., lack of use of
a limb), neurological symptoms (e.g., presence of spasticity*), and physical limitations (e.g., delayed independent sitting or walking). However,

---

* A condition in which there is an abnormal increase in muscle tone or stiffness of muscle that can
interfere with movement and speech, and be associated with discomfort or pain.[22]

using certain standardized tests in combination with clinical examination and medical history, Novak and colleagues found that a diagnosis of CP can often accurately be made before six months corrected age.[*][21] They identified two distinct pathways in their International Clinical Practice Guideline for early diagnosis of CP:

- Before five months corrected age, for infants with newborn detectable risk factors (e.g., preterm):
  ○ MRI (magnetic resonance imaging)
  ○ GMs (Prechtl Qualitative Assessment of General Movements)[†]
  ○ HINE (Hammersmith Infant Neurological Examination)[‡]
- After five months corrected age for infants with infant detectable risk factors (e.g., delayed motor milestones)
  ○ MRI
  ○ HINE
  ○ DAYC (Developmental Assessment of Young Children)[§]

The presence of a brain injury is confirmed by MRI in many but not all children with CP. Imaging may also help determine when the brain injury occurred.[3] However, up to 17 percent of children diagnosed with CP have normal MRI brain scans.[3] For these children, best practice is to investigate further to rule out genetic and metabolic conditions.[3]

Successful implementation of early diagnosis programs has been demonstrated in different countries.[23-28] Early diagnosis is very important because it allows for early intervention, which helps to achieve better functional outcomes for the child.

---

* The term "corrected age" refers to how old an infant would be if they had been born on their due date rather than preterm. "Chronological age" refers to how old an infant is from their date of birth. Corrected age is often used when assessing growth and developmental skills usually up to a chronological age of two years. With preterm infants, it takes time to determine whether the delays are related to being preterm or are true delays.

† A standardized assessment of movement for infants, from birth to five months corrected age. It involves a video of an infant lying on their back while they are awake, calm, and alert. The recorded movements are then scored by a certified medical professional.

‡ A standardized neurological examination for infants age 2 to 24 months performed by a medical professional. There are three parts to the exam: carrying out a neurological examination (which is scored), noting developmental milestones, and observing behavior (both not scored).

§ A standardized assessment for infants and children from birth to five years, in which a medical professional scores a child's skills during observation of play or daily activity, asking a child to perform a skill, or by interviewing parents to measure ability in five domains: cognition, communication, social-emotional development, physical development, and adaptive behavior.

Where a CP diagnosis is suspected but cannot be made with certainty, using the interim diagnosis of "high risk for CP" is recommended until a diagnosis is confirmed.[29] This allows the child to receive the benefits of CP-specific early intervention.[30]

These early interventions are designed to:[21]

- Optimize motor, cognition, and communication skills using interventions that promote learning and neuroplasticity
- Prevent secondary impairments and minimize complications that worsen function or interfere with learning (e.g., monitor hips, control epilepsy, take care of sleeping, feeding)
- Promote parent or caregiver coping and mental health

Neuroplasticity (also known as brain plasticity, neural plasticity, and neuronal plasticity) refers to the brain's ability to change. After a brain injury occurs, the brain will try to recover somewhat by creating new pathways around the injury, moving functions to a healthy area of the brain, or strengthening existing healthy connections. This potential for change and growth through practice and repetition allows the brain to develop new skills.[31,32]

Neuroplasticity is at its optimum during early brain development. The first thousand days are a critical time for brain development; this is a time when interventions are particularly effective.[33] This is also a time of extreme vulnerability: the same neuroplasticity that gives a child the potential to recover function also makes them very sensitive to any intervention, which can result in unwanted consequences unless the intervention has been proven safe.

Morgan and colleagues published an International Clinical Practice Guideline for early intervention for children from birth to two years of age with or at high risk of CP.[30] They followed this with another guideline in 2023 for children in the first year of life, which helps determine the most appropriate motor intervention to implement.[34]

These clinical practice guidelines for early diagnosis and early intervention should become standard of care[21,30,34] and be continually updated. The advancements in early diagnosis have resulted in multiple clinical trials in early interventions around the world, which will add to the research base in the coming years. (Further information on clinical trials is included in Chapter 11.)

Graham and colleagues noted that mothers of children with CP who have previously had a typically developing child often sense that something is wrong at a very early stage; they advised professionals to take the concerns of an experienced parent seriously.[3] Indeed, "parent-identified concern" is included in the International Clinical Practice Guideline for early diagnosis as a "valid reason to trigger formal diagnostic investigations and referral to early intervention."[21] Parent focus groups have also found that receiving early diagnosis or high risk for CP classification is a parent priority.[35]

Emily Perl Kingsley, who was a writer on the TV show *Sesame Street*, wrote a short essay titled "Welcome to Holland" in 1987 about parenting her son, born with Down syndrome. She described it as going on vacation and arriving at a different destination than what was expected. The essay resonates with many families on receiving a diagnosis of CP and is included in **Useful web resources**.

I feel it would be a disservice to not make note of the impact that a diagnosis of CP has on a family, especially the mother, but also the father, siblings, and extended family. I felt overwhelmed with guilt and sorrow when my children were born prematurely. That guilt compounded as Levi's needs became clearer and he was unable to do the things his brother could do. That guilt and stress factored into the dissolution over time of my marriage to Levi's father and would become a foundational part of what would eventually become my C-PTSD (complex post-traumatic stress disorder).

Nobody warns you that your child being diagnosed with a serious disease or condition will impact you as well. I think if I had known the level of stress and guilt that would come with a diagnosis and been told to take care of my own mental health, I would have been more intentional about self-care and relationship care. The number of parents who leave the NICU with their own trauma and PTSD is scarily high, and while a forewarning is not prevention, I believe it would have been helpful.

My suggestion to any parent hearing their child's diagnosis of spastic quadriplegic CP is to put your own mental health at the forefront. Your child has a long, winding road ahead of them, but so do you. Being a special needs parent is hard. It is stressful. There will be days where you don't recognize yourself in the mirror, and nights spent sleeping in hospitals. You will hear friends, family, and complete strangers say to you, "I don't know how you do it." Your response will be, "Some days I don't know either, but with love and faith anything is possible!"

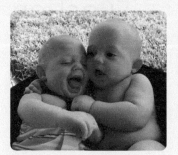

Levi (left) and Cam (right).

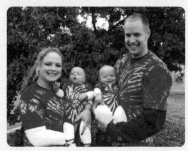

Mom (Kate) holding Levi, and Dad (Chris) holding Cam.

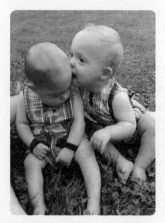

Levi (left) and Cam (right).

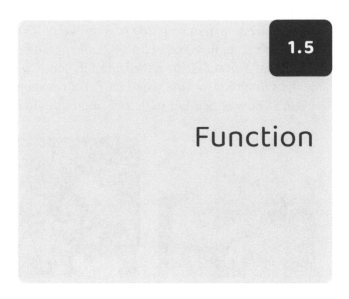

Function

That's one small step for man, one giant leap for mankind.

Neil Armstrong

"Function" means ability or capacity. "Motor function" refers to our ability to move, and "communication function" refers to our ability to transmit and receive information by whatever means. CP affects the development of movement, but it can also affect other areas, such as cognition. This section introduces the broad area of function and, again, lays groundwork for later sections.

Developmental milestones

The CDC published a series of developmental milestones that address typical development of the child from the age of two months to five years, in the following areas:[36]

- Social/emotional
- Language/communication

- Cognitive
- Movement/physical development

These milestones are an important reference when a child appears to be late in development compared with typically developing children. The CDC developmental milestones are included in **Useful web resources**.

Movement and physical development depend on the development and maturation of gross and fine motor function.

- **Gross motor function** (or gross motor skills): the movement of the arms, legs, and other large body parts. It involves the use of large muscles. Examples include sitting, crawling, standing, running, jumping, swimming, throwing, catching, and kicking. These movements involve maintaining balance and changing position.
- **Fine motor function** (or fine motor skills, hand skills, fine motor coordination, or dexterity): the smaller movements that occur in the wrists, hands, fingers, feet, and toes. It involves the control of small muscles. Examples include picking up objects between the thumb and forefinger, and writing. These movements typically involve hand-eye coordination and require a high degree of precision of hand and finger movement.

There is a usual sequence and timing to the achievement of gross motor developmental milestones in the typically developing child. A large study conducted by the World Health Organization (WHO) found that, with some variation, almost all typically developing children have achieved independent sitting by 9 months and independent walking by 18 months.[37] The average age and age range for achieving each of six gross motor developmental milestones are shown in Figure 1.5.1.

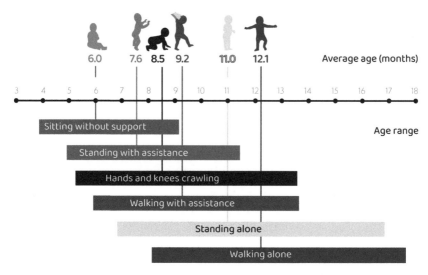

Figure 1.5.1 Average age and age range of gross motor developmental milestones.

The earlier motor development stages—sitting, standing, and sometimes, crawling—are important for the development of walking. Developmental stages build on each other. Early milestones in most cases are prerequisites to later ones, with crawling being the exception as not all children crawl.[37]

Milestones are an important reference when a child appears to be late in development compared with typically developing children. For example, one of the hallmarks of CP is that the child may be late or never achieve gross motor developmental milestones. In fact, that may be what first alerts parents or professionals to a problem. It is important to acknowledge that this can be a point of grieving for families.

The development of function is under the control of the nervous system and is affected to varying degrees in CP. Function may improve somewhat without treatment, but treatment is essential to maximize function as early as possible, which is why early intervention is so important.

Measuring function

A number of standardized measurement (assessment) tools may be used to measure function. Examples include:

- DAYC (Developmental Assessment of Young Children) for infants and children from birth to five years
- Peabody Developmental Motor Scales for infants and children from birth to five years
- Bayley Scales of Infant and Toddler Development for infants and children from 1 to 42 months
- Gross Motor Function Measure (GMFM) for children with CP aged five months to 16 years.

Information on these and other measurement tools is included in Appendix 1 (online).

Because I had been told that Levi's PVL would likely result in some form of CP, I knew that his developmental milestones would be affected. Because he had an identical twin who did not have PVL, I had a sort of "norm" to which I could compare his delays. I knew that every child develops at their own pace, but I felt I could roughly compare the twins and get an idea of just how far "behind" Levi was. I would come to learn, over time, that this comparison was not only unhelpful, it was also unhealthy for me and my boys. It gave me unrealistic expectations and prevented me from celebrating the child I had. There is also a freedom in accepting your child for who they are in the moment.

Over the first two years of their lives, Cam grew up to meet his normal developmental milestones of rolling over, sitting up, walking, and talking, and his brother just didn't. By the time Levi was about two years old, we knew that the doctor's prediction of "tightness in his ankles" was a very optimistic view of what the PVL and CP had done to his body.

Because the twins were born at 27 weeks, they qualified for special education services from the get-go. They both received physical therapy (PT), occupational therapy (OT), and eventually speech therapy starting at birth and continuing until they were five years old. At age five, Levi continued to qualify for school-based special education services, while his brother aged out.

Because Levi was quite sick during his first few years of life (he had 13 surgeries or procedures in his first year), I didn't have time to wrap my head around much else besides hospital stays. I didn't know that he should have been receiving additional private therapy, but by the time he turned three, I had him in private sessions of PT, OT, and speech therapy. I highly suggest doubling up on therapies as soon as possible (school or county based, and private).

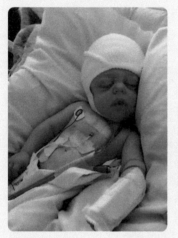 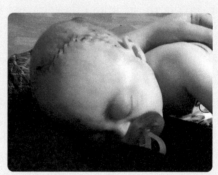

Levi after surgery at age six months.

Classification based on predominant motor type and topography

Order and simplification are the first steps toward the mastery of a subject—the actual enemy is the unknown.
Thomas Mann

Over the years, there has been much discussion of the classification of CP. Classification, or dividing into groups, is useful because it provides information about the nature of the condition and its severity (its level or magnitude). It also allows us to learn from people who have the condition at a similar level.

This section addresses classification of CP based on predominant motor type and topography. ("Predominant motor type" means the predominant abnormal muscle tone* and movement impairment, and "topography" means area of the body affected.) It also covers location of the brain injury and prevalence of CP by subtype. The next section looks at classification of CP based on functional ability.

---

* The resting tension in a person's muscles. A range of normal muscle tone exists. Tone is considered abnormal when it falls outside the range of normal or typical. It can be too low (hypotonia) or too high (hypertonia).

CP subtype based on predominant motor type

There are several subtypes of CP based on the predominant motor type. These include:

- Spasticity—spastic CP
- Dyskinesia—dyskinetic CP
- Ataxia—ataxic CP
- Hypotonia—hypotonic CP[4]

See Table 1.6.1.

Table 1.6.1 CP subtypes based on predominant motor type

CP SUBTYPE	EXPLANATION
Spasticity—spastic CP	Spasticity is a condition in which there is an abnormal increase in muscle tone or stiffness of muscle that can interfere with movement and speech, and be associated with discomfort or pain.[22]
Dyskinesia—dyskinetic CP	Dyskinesia is a condition in which there are "abnormal patterns of posture and/or movement associated with involuntary, uncontrolled, recurring, occasionally stereotyped movement patterns."[8] ("Stereotyped movement patterns" means the movements are in a particular pattern, specific to that person, which is repeated.) Dyskinetic CP can be subdivided into either dystonic or choreo-athetotic CP.[38] • **Dystonic (dystonia):** Dystonia is characterized by involuntary (unintended) muscle contractions that cause slow repetitive movements or abnormal postures that can sometimes be painful.[39] • **Choreo-athetotic (choreo-athetosis):** ○ Chorea is characterized by jerky, dance-like movements.[3] ○ Athetosis is characterized by slow, writhing movements.[3]

Cont'd.

CP SUBTYPE	EXPLANATION
Ataxia—ataxic CP	Ataxia means "without coordination." People with ataxic CP "experience a failure of muscle control in their arms and legs, resulting in a lack of balance and coordination or a disturbance of gait."[40]
Hypotonia—hypotonic CP	Hypotonia is a condition in which there is an abnormal decrease in muscle tone.[22] The muscles are floppy.

It is worth noting that these abnormal muscle tone or movement impairments may be present in other conditions, not just CP.

CP subtype based on topography

There are two methods of classifying CP subtypes based on topography. One is older (historical), and one has been more recently adopted (SCPE).

With the first method, the names of all the subtypes have the suffix "plegia," which is derived from the Greek word for stroke, although there are causes of CP other than a stroke. The prefixes in the names of the subtypes—"mono," "hemi," "di," "tri," and "quad," also derived from Greek, or Latin—indicate how many limbs are affected (see Table 1.6.2).*

---

* Occasionally, the terms "hemiparesis" for spastic hemiplegia, "diparesis" for spastic diplegia, and "quadriparesis" for spastic quadriplegia are used.[41]

Table 1.6.2 CP subtypes based on topography—historical

CP SUBTYPE	AREA OF BODY AFFECTED	
Monoplegia		Mono = One. One limb, usually one of the lower limbs.
Hemiplegia		Hemi = Half. Upper and lower limbs on one side of the body. The upper limb is usually more affected than the lower limb.
Diplegia		Di = Two. All limbs, but the lower limbs much more than the upper ones, which frequently show only fine motor impairment.
Triplegia		Tri = Three. Three limbs, usually the two lower limbs and one upper limb. The lower limb on the side of the upper limb involvement is usually more affected.
Quadriplegia		Quad = Four. All four limbs and the trunk; also known as tetraplegia.

One of the disadvantages of the historical classification system is a lack of precision.[8] However, this system has been and continues to be used extensively, particularly in the US.

The Surveillance of Cerebral Palsy in Europe network (SCPE) has developed a simpler classification method, also based on topography.[38] This method is now generally used in Europe and Australia. It identifies two main subtypes of CP: unilateral and bilateral (see Table 1.6.3).

Table 1.6.3 CP subtypes based on topography—SCPE

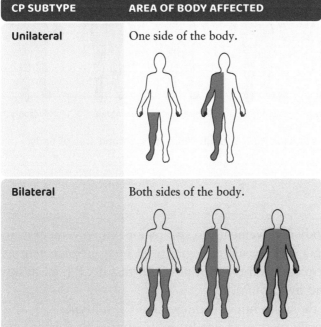

CP SUBTYPE	AREA OF BODY AFFECTED
Unilateral	One side of the body.
Bilateral	Both sides of the body.

Location of brain injury

Different subtypes of CP result from injury to different parts of the brain:

- Spasticity is associated with injury to the cerebrum.
- Dyskinesia is associated with injury to the basal ganglia and thalamus.
- Ataxia is associated with injury to the cerebellum.
- Hypotonia is associated with injury to the cerebrum and cerebellum.

Figure 1.6.1 summarizes CP subtypes, predominant motor types, topography, and location of brain injury.

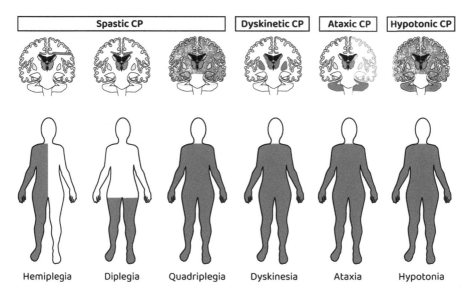

Figure 1.6.1 CP subtypes and location of brain injury (orange) and area of body affected (green).

Figure 1.6.1 shows:

- The extent of body involvement (green): regional involvement as in spastic hemiplegia and spastic diplegia; total body involvement as in spastic quadriplegia and the nonspastic forms of CP (i.e., dyskinesia, ataxia, and hypotonia).
- The location of the brain injury (orange) and CP subtype:
  - Injury primarily to the left cerebrum causing right side spastic hemiplegia (and vice versa)
  - Injury to both left and right cerebrum causing spastic diplegia
  - More extensive injury to both left and right cerebrum causing spastic quadriplegia
  - Injury to the basal ganglia and thalamus causing dyskinesia
  - Injury to the cerebellum causing ataxia
  - Injury to both left and right cerebrum and cerebellum causing hypotonia

Note that this is a *very* simplified explanation. In reality, CP is much more nuanced. For example, there may be more than one area of brain injury. In addition, particularly with a preterm birth, brain injury may happen more than once. As well, the brain injury can vary from very mild to very severe.

Knowledge of the brain injury sometimes confirms the symptoms seen in a child. MRI scans are becoming more routine with CP. However, up to 17 percent of children with CP have normal MRI brain scans.[3]

Recall that the brain injury in CP is unchanging (i.e., the size and location do not change), but "unchanging" may be a bit misleading since with time, growth, and maturation of the brain and other structures, the effects of the brain injury become more apparent in the form of motor delays and problems with other body systems.

Prevalence of CP by subtype

Figure 1.6.2 shows the prevalence of CP by predominant motor type and topography for almost 11,000 Australian children with CP.[4,42] While precise percentages of prevalence are different in other countries, the data in Figure 1.6.2 is from a large dataset and is consistent with studies from other countries.[43–46] It shows that:

- The predominant motor type is spastic (78 percent).
- Hemiplegia, diplegia, and quadriplegia each represent approximately one-third of the total.

Note that only spastic CP is subdivided by topography because the other subtypes (i.e., dyskinetic, ataxic, and hypotonic CP) generally affect the whole body.

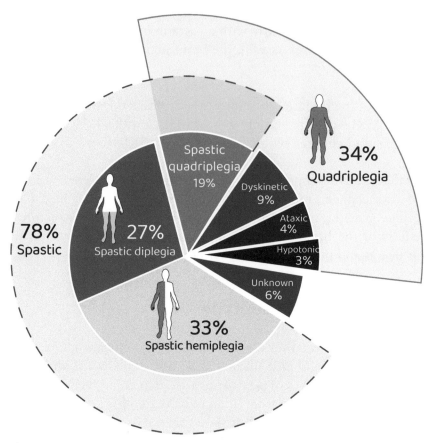

Figure 1.6.2 Predominant motor type and topography for Australian children with CP.[4,42]

It is important to note that different CP registers regard hypotonia differently. The Australian CP register includes hypotonia as a subtype of CP; the European CP register does not. Figure 1.6.2 shows that 3 percent of Australian children with CP were classified as having hypotonic CP.[4] One study found that only 46 percent of physicians who diagnose CP in the US and Canada would diagnose it in the case of hypotonia.[47] A diagnosis of CP is important because it may affect access to rehabilitation services in some countries.

Finally, it's important to understand that while CP is classified based on the predominant motor type, many individuals have secondary or co-occurring motor types. Data from the Australian CP register, for example, showed that 48 percent of individuals with spastic quadriplegia have co-occurring dyskinesia, and it is believed that the true prevalence of co-occurring motor types is higher.[4] A more recent report found that 50 percent of children and young people with CP had spasticity and dystonia.[48]

The co-occurrence of dystonia with spasticity has been underrecognized. This is important to know because management of spasticity and management of dystonia are different.

Classification based on functional ability

It is our choices, Harry, that show what we truly are,
far more than our abilities.

J.K. Rowling

A series of functional ability classification systems has been developed, with each having the same structure and common language. These systems include classifying CP based on:

- Functional mobility (as in movement from place to place)
- Manual ability (ability to handle objects)
- Communication ability
- Eating and drinking ability
- Visual function

Functional mobility

The Gross Motor Function Classification System (GMFCS) is a five-level classification system that describes the functional mobility of children and adolescents with CP.[49] The GMFCS and the expanded, revised version—GMFCS E&R[50]—includes descriptions for five age groups:

- 0 to 2 years
- 2 to 4 years
- 4 to 6 years
- 6 to 12 years
- 12 to 18 years

The emphasis is on the child's or adolescent's usual performance in their daily environment (i.e., their home and community).[*] By choosing which description best matches the child at their current age, they can be assigned a GMFCS level.

Table 1.7.1 describes the five levels. The severity of the movement limitations increases with each level, with level I having the fewest movement limitations and level V having the most. It is important to note, however, that the differences between the levels are not equal.

Table 1.7.1 Functional mobility across the five levels of the GMFCS[49,50]

GMFCS LEVEL	FUNCTIONAL MOBILITY
I	Walks without limitations
II	Walks with limitations
III	Walks using a handheld mobility device (assistive walking device)[*]
IV	Self-mobility with limitations; may use powered mobility[†]
V	Transported in a manual wheelchair

[*] Handheld mobility device (assistive walking device) includes canes, crutches, and walkers that do not support the weight of the trunk during walking.

[†] Powered mobility includes wheelchairs and scooters controlled by a joystick or electrical switch.

---

[*] In this context, "community" may be interpreted as "away from home." Moving about at home is generally easier since it is likely well suited or adapted to the person's needs. The community may be more challenging. It is important to keep in mind the impact of environmental and personal factors on what children and adolescents are able to do in their daily environment (home or community). See section 1.8, The International Classification of Functioning, Disability and Health.

The GMFCS levels are based on the method of functional mobility that best describes the child's performance after age six, but a child can be classified much earlier using these descriptions. They are relatively stable after age two.[49,51,52] In fact, stability into young adulthood has been demonstrated. McCormick and colleagues found that a GMFCS level observed around age 12 was highly predictive of motor function in early adulthood.[53]

Knowing a child's level offers insight into what the future may hold in terms of their mobility. It helps answer some of the many questions parents may have in the early days, such as, "Will my child walk?" or, "How serious is their CP?"

The full version of the GMFCS E&R is a short document and is included in **Useful web resources**. It contains further detail on functional mobility for each age and GMFCS level. It also includes a summary of the distinctions between each level to help determine which level most closely resembles a particular child's or adolescent's functional mobility. Useful illustrations have been developed based on the GMFCS for the two upper age bands (6 to 12 years and 12 to 18 years) by staff at the Royal Children's Hospital in Melbourne (see Figures 1.7.1 and 1.7.2).

GMFCS E & R between 6th and 12th birthday: Descriptors and illustrations

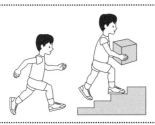

GMFCS Level I

Children walk at home, school, outdoors and in the community. They can climb stairs without the use of a railing. Children perform gross motor skills such as running and jumping, but speed, balance and coordination are limited.

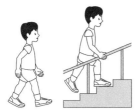

GMFCS Level II

Children walk in most settings and climb stairs holding onto a railing. They may experience difficulty walking long distances and balancing on uneven terrain, inclines, in crowded areas or confined spaces. Children may walk with physical assistance, a hand-held mobility device or used wheeled mobility over long distances. Children have only minimal ability to perform gross motor skills such as running and jumping.

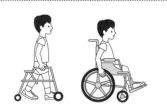

GMFCS Level III

Children walk using a hand-held mobility device in most indoor settings. They may climb stairs holding onto a railing with supervision or assistance. Children use wheeled mobility when traveling long distances and may self-propel for shorter distances.

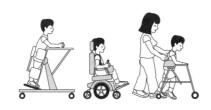

GMFCS Level IV

Children use methods of mobility that require physical assistance or powered mobility in most settings. They may walk for short distances at home with physical assistance or use powered mobility or a body support walker when positioned. At school, outdoors and in the community children are transported in a manual wheelchair or use powered mobility.

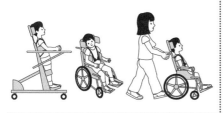

GMFCS Level V

Children are transported in a manual wheelchair in all settings. Children are limited in their ability to maintain antigravity head and trunk postures and control leg and arm movements.

GMFCS descriptors: Palisano et al. (1997) Dev Med Child Neurol 39:214-23
CanChild: www.canchild.ca

Illustrations Version 2 © Bill Reid, Kate Willoughby, Adrienne Harvey and Kerr Graham, The Royal Children's Hospital Melbourne ERC151050

Figure 1.7.1 GMFCS E&R between 6th and 12th birthday: Descriptors and illustrations. Reproduced with kind permission from K. Graham and K. Willoughby, Royal Children's Hospital Melbourne, Australia.

GMFCS E & R between 12th and 18th birthday: Descriptors and illustrations

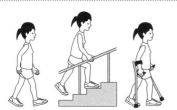

GMFCS Level I

Youth walk at home, school, outdoors and in the community. Youth are able to climb curbs and stairs without physical assistance or a railing. They perform gross motor skills such as running and jumping but speed, balance and coordination are limited.

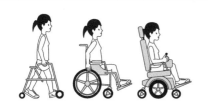

GMFCS Level II

Youth walk in most settings but environmental factors and personal choice influence mobility choices. At school or work they may require a hand held mobility device for safety and climb stairs holding onto a railing. Outdoors and in the community youth may use wheeled mobility when traveling long distances.

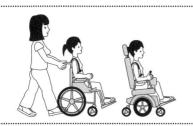

GMFCS Level III

Youth are capable of walking using a hand-held mobility device. Youth may climb stairs holding onto a railing with supervision or assistance. At school they may self-propel a manual wheelchair or use powered mobility. Outdoors and in the community youth are transported in a wheelchair or use powered mobility.

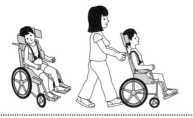

GMFCS Level IV

Youth use wheeled mobility in most settings. Physical assistance of 1-2 people is required for transfers. Indoors, youth may walk short distances with physical assistance, use wheeled mobility or a body support walker when positioned. They may operate a powered chair, otherwise are transported in a manual wheelchair.

GMFCS Level V

Youth are transported in a manual wheelchair in all settings. Youth are limited in their ability to maintain antigravity head and trunk postures and control leg and arm movements. Self-mobility is severely limited, even with the use of assistive technology.

GMFCS descriptors: Palisano et al. (1997) Dev Med Child Neurol 39:214-23
CanChild: www.canchild.ca

Illustrations Version 2 © Bill Reid, Kate Willoughby, Adrienne Harvey and Kerr Graham, The Royal Children's Hospital Melbourne ERC151050

Figure 1.7.2 GMFCS E&R between 12th and 18th birthday: Descriptors and illustrations. Reproduced with kind permission from K. Graham and K. Willoughby, Royal Children's Hospital Melbourne, Australia.

One use of the GMFCS has been classifying walking ability into three levels:[54]

- **Mild:** independent walker; GMFCS levels I–II
- **Moderate:** walker with aid; GMFCS level III
- **Severe:** wheelchair; GMFCS levels IV–V

In addition, the GMFCS led to the development of the gross motor development curves.[55,56] The curves show the change in gross motor function over time as measured by the Gross Motor Function Measure-66 (GMFM-66).* There are five curves, one for each GMFCS level (see Figure 1.7.3).

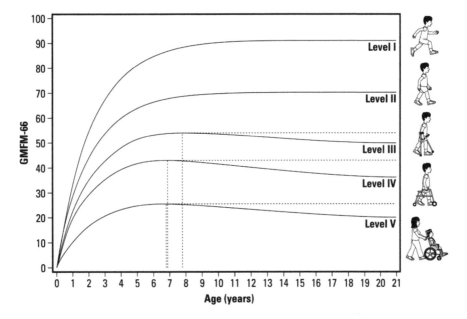

Figure 1.7.3 Gross motor curves in children with CP and the five levels of the GMFCS. Adapted with kind permission from *Cerebral Palsy: Science and Clinical Practice*, edited by B. Dan et al. (2014). Mac Keith Press.

The curves allow us to see how a child's gross motor function is likely to develop over time, as measured by the GMFM-66. The figure shows

---

* A standardized assessment tool used to evaluate the gross motor function of individuals with CP. It consists of 66 items that assess a wide range of gross motor skills. Also used is GMFM-88, which assesses 88 items. Each addresses five areas of increasing gross motor function: 1) lying and rolling, 2) sitting, 3) crawling and kneeling, 4) standing, and 5) walking, running, and jumping.

the average GMFM-66 score (vertical y-axis) at each GMFCS level by age (horizontal x-axis). Specifically, it shows:

- For each level there is an initial rapid rise in score to a peak, then it plateaus (levels I–II) or decreases (levels III–V).
- The score is highest for level I and lowest for level V.
- The dotted lines show the age at which the score peaks and the decrease from the peak to age 21 years for levels III–V (the oldest participants in the study were 21, so the shape of the curves after 21 are not known).
- Even a child at level I does not reach 100, the maximum, on the scale.

These curves are based on averages, and it is important to remember that some children were above and some below the line at each level.[55] Still, they are very useful. Why? Because they help answer some of the many questions parents have in the early days. Knowing a child's GMFCS level at age two, for example, allows parents to see how the child's gross motor function, as measured by the GMFM-66, is likely to develop over time. However, it is worth noting that the curves are not accurate before the age of two.

While remaining very realistic in expectations, the focus should be on helping the child reach their maximum possible gross motor function, not just hitting the average. The curves should guide, but not limit, a child's potential.

As Levi and his twin brother grew into toddlers, their differences became glaringly obvious. Cam was sitting up, crawling, and eventually walking on his own, while Levi was unable to do any of those things unassisted. For many years, Levi could take steps with a gait trainer* or when being held by an adult; however, as he got bigger, he was not able to hold his weight in a walking stance. In those early days, it was a joy to see Cam meeting his milestones, but that joy compounded the sadness of seeing Levi not making the same progress. Because Levi was

---

* A walker that offers increased postural support, weight-bearing capabilities, and mobility assistance while walking.

in so many therapies, I held on to the hope that one day he would walk, though it may look different or need a device like a gait trainer.

When your child has spastic quad CP, statistics can be discouraging. Children with GMFCS V spastic quad CP do not walk independently, and it became clear when Levi was about three or four that would be his future. I am very glad that I had him in so many therapies, as the time spent working muscles and practicing movements was invaluable.

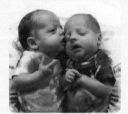

Cam (left) and Levi (right).

Manual ability

The Manual Ability Classification System (MACS) is a five-level classification system that describes how children and adolescents with CP age 4 to 18 years handle objects in daily activities.[57] The levels are based on the individual's ability to handle objects (relevant and age appropriate) and their need for assistance or adaptation. A separate Mini-MACS is available for children age one to four.[58]

Table 1.7.2 describes the five levels. Limitations of manual ability increase with increasing MACS level. As with the GMFCS, the differences between levels are not equal. The scale is used to classify overall ability to handle objects, *not* each hand separately. The emphasis is on the child's or adolescent's overall usual performance in their daily environment (their home, school, and community), rather than what is known to be their best performance.

Table 1.7.2 Ability to handle objects across the five levels of the MACS[57]

MACS LEVEL	ABILITY TO HANDLE OBJECTS
I	Handles objects easily and successfully
II	Handles most objects but with somewhat reduced quality and/or speed of achievement
III	Handles objects with difficulty; needs help to prepare and/or modify activities
IV	Handles a limited selection of easily managed objects in adapted situations
V	Does not handle objects and has severely limited ability to perform even simple actions

The full versions of the MACS and Mini-MACS are short documents and are included in **Useful web resources**. They provide further detail on each level and a summary of the distinctions between adjacent levels to help determine the most appropriate level for the individual.

An alternative to the MACS is the Bimanual Fine Motor Function (BFMF)[59,60,61] (see Figure 1.7.4). Unlike the MACS (and Mini-MACS), the BFMF assesses the child's ability to grasp, hold, and manipulate objects in *each* hand separately.[60] More information on the BFMF is included in **Useful web resources.**

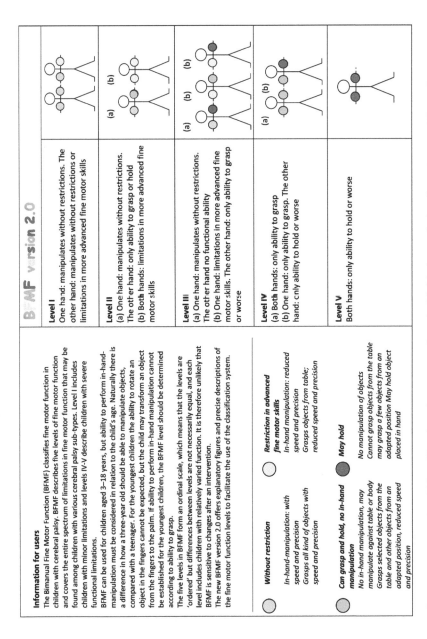

Information for users

The Bimanual Fine Motor Function (BFMF) classifies fine motor function in children with cerebral palsy. BFMF describes five levels of limitations in fine motor function and covers the entire spectrum of limitations in fine motor function that may be found among children with various cerebral palsy sub-types. Level I includes children with minor limitations and levels IV–V describe children with severe functional limitations.

BFMF can be used for children aged 3–18 years, but ability to perform in-hand-manipulation must be considered in relation to the child's age. Naturally there is a difference in how a three-year old should be able to manipulate objects, compared with a teenager. For the youngest children the ability to rotate an object in the fingers cannot be expected, but the child may transform an object from the fingers to the palm. If ability to perform in-hand manipulation cannot be established for the youngest children, the BFMF level should be determined according to ability to grasp.

The five levels in BFMF form an ordinal scale, which means that the levels are 'ordered' but differences between levels are not necessarily equal, and each level includes children with relatively varied function. It is therefore unlikely that BFMF is sensitive to changes after an intervention.

The new BFMF version 2.0 offers explanatory figures and precise descriptions of the fine motor function levels to facilitate the use of the classification system.

○ *Without restriction*

In-hand-manipulation: with speed and precision
Grasps all kind of objects with speed and precision

○ *Restriction in advanced fine motor skills*

In-hand manipulation: reduced speed and precision
Grasps objects from table; reduced speed and precision

● *Can grasp and hold, no in-hand manipulation*

No in-hand manipulation, may manipulate against table or body
Grasps selected objects from the table and other objects from an adapted position, reduced speed and precision

● *May hold*

No manipulation of objects
Cannot grasp objects from the table
may grasp a few objects from an adapted position May hold object placed in hand

BFMF version 2.0

Level I
One hand: manipulates without restrictions. The other hand: manipulates without restrictions or limitations in more advanced fine motor skills

Level II
(a) One hand: manipulates without restrictions. The other hand: only ability to grasp or hold
(b) Both hands: limitations in more advanced fine motor skills

Level III
(a) One hand: manipulates without restrictions. The other hand no functional ability
(b) One hand: limitations in more advanced fine motor skills. The other hand: only ability to grasp or worse

Level IV
(a) Both hands: only ability to grasp
(b) One hand: only ability to grasp. The other hand: only ability to hold or worse

Level V
Both hands: only ability to hold or worse

Figure 1.7.4 BFMF level identification chart. Reproduced with kind permission from Dr. Kate Himmelmann and Dr. Ann-Kristin Elvrum.

Communication ability

The Communication Function Classification System (CFCS) is a five-level classification system that describes everyday communication performance for children with CP.[62] Table 1.7.3 describes the five levels. Hidecker and colleagues have defined some key concepts used in this classification system:

> *Communication occurs when a **sender** transmits a message, **and** a **receiver** understands the message ... **Unfamiliar conversational partners** are strangers or acquaintances who only occasionally communicate with the person. **Familiar conversational partners** such as relatives, caregivers, and friends may be able to communicate more effectively with the person because of previous knowledge and personal experiences ... All methods of communication performance are considered ... These include speech, gestures, behaviors, eye gaze, facial expressions, and augmentative and alternative communication (AAC).[62]*

Table 1.7.3 Communication ability across the five levels of the CFCS[62]

CFCS LEVEL	COMMUNICATION ABILITY
I	Effective sender and receiver with unfamiliar and familiar partners
II	Effective but slower-paced sender and/or receiver with unfamiliar and/or familiar partners
III	Effective sender and receiver with familiar partners
IV	Inconsistent sender and/or receiver with familiar partners
V	Seldom-effective sender and receiver even with familiar partners

An alternative to the CFCS is the Viking Speech Scale (VSS),[63,64,65] but it addresses just speech. It is a four-point scale, with level I having the fewest limitations and level IV the most (see Table 1.7.4).

Table 1.7.4 Viking Speech Scale

VSS LEVEL	SPEECH UNDERSTANDABILITY
I	Speech is not affected by motor disorder.
II	Speech is imprecise but usually understandable to unfamiliar listeners.
III	Speech is unclear and not usually understandable to unfamiliar listeners out of context.
IV	No understandable speech.

More information on both the CFCS and VSS is included in **Useful web resources.**

Levi has perfected the art of nonverbal communication and manipulation. I would place him at a IV or V on the CFCS. He makes different types of laughs, cries, and noises that are understood by people who are familiar with him. We believe that Levi also understands what we are saying to him, though he has a slower processing time when he is trying to make his body react to a question. For example, if I tell Levi to smile if he wants to go outside, he needs 30 seconds or more to get his body to smile. He also needs this time to activate buttons or use his eye gaze as well.

Eating and drinking ability

The Eating and Drinking Ability Classification System (EDACS) is used for individuals with CP who are age three and older.[66] The EDACS assesses eating and drinking from two perspectives across the five levels:[66]

- **Safety:** For example, aspiration (food or liquid entering the airway or lungs instead of the esophagus) and choking (blockage of the airway by food)
- **Efficiency:** Amount of food and liquid lost from the mouth and time taken to eat

Table 1.7.5 describes the five levels.

Table 1.7.5 Eating and drinking ability across the five levels of the EDACS[66]

EDACS LEVEL	EATING AND DRINKING ABILITY
I	Eats and drinks safely and efficiently
II	Eats and drinks safely but with some limitations to efficiency
III	Eats and drinks with some limitations to safety; there may be limitations to efficiency
IV	Eats and drinks with significant limitations to safety
V	Unable to eat and drink safely—tube-feeding may be considered to provide nutrition

Useful illustrations for the EDACS from age three years have been developed focusing on the safety and efficiency aspects of feeding (see Figure 1.7.5).

Levi is EDACS level V. Levi was a pretty good eater until he got sick when he was about 18 months old, though he did often projectile vomit after eating. Somehow, he contracted *Salmonella* Paratyphi infection, usually found in Southeast Asia. We are still confused about how that happened. While in the hospital with a fever of 106.8 °F, he stopped taking liquid by mouth. He was still eating baby foods though. After a few days, we were told he needed a feeding tube, but we could continue to feed Levi by mouth and just use the tube for liquids overnight if needed.

What we didn't know at the time is that having a feeding tube may cause a child to lose interest in eating by mouth, which is exactly what happened with Levi. We learned that the hard way, and after a few years of focusing on feeding therapy, we conceded that Levi would simply be 100 percent tube-fed.

When making decisions about your child's care, it's important to make sure they are informed decisions. I strongly recommend doing your homework to understand procedures. And be sure to ask questions, too.

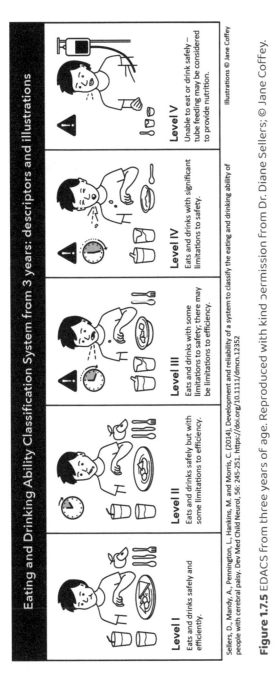

Eating and Drinking Ability Classification System from 3 years: descriptors and illustrations

Level I
Eats and drinks safely and efficiently.

Level II
Eats and drinks safely but with some limitations to efficiency.

Level III
Eats and drinks with some limitations to safety; there may be limitations to efficiency.

Level IV
Eats and drinks with significant limitations to safety.

Level V
Unable to eat or drink safely – tube feeding may be considered to provide nutrition.

Sellers, D., Mandy, A., Pennington, L., Hankins, M. and Morris, C. (2014). Development and reliability of a system to classify the eating and drinking ability of people with cerebral palsy. Dev Med Child Neurol, 56: 245-251. https://doi.org/10.1111/dmcn.12352

Illustrations © Jane Coffey

Figure 1.7.5 EDACS from three years of age. Reproduced with kind permission from Dr. Diane Sellers; © Jane Coffey.

A Mini-EDACS has been developed for children with CP from age 18 to 36 months.[67] More information on the EDACS and Mini-EDACS is included in **Useful web resources.**

Visual function

The Visual Function Classification System (VFCS) is for individuals with CP from the age of one. Table 1.7.6 describes the five levels.

Table 1.7.6 Visual function across the five levels of the VFCS[68]

VFCS LEVEL	VISUAL FUNCTION
I	Uses visual function easily and successfully in vision-related activities
II	Uses visual function successfully but needs self-initiated compensatory strategies
III	Uses visual function but needs some adaptations
IV	Uses visual function in very adapted environments but performs just part of vision-related activities
V	Does not use visual function even in very adapted environments

More information on the VFCS is included in **Useful web resources.**

Using classification systems

Together, the various classification systems provide a lot of information, and each is valid and reliable.[*,68,69] Because families can understand (and assign) classification system levels,[69,70] the systems can help with communication between medical professionals and families. They also help with good planning of care both in the present and into the future since

---

* A good classification system must be:
  • **Valid:** It measures what it claims to measure.
  • **Reliable:** It provides the same answer when used by different people or by the same person at different times.
  • **Accurate:** It measures how close a value is to its true value (e.g., how close an arrow gets to the target).
  • **Precise:** It measures how repeatable a measurement is (e.g., how close the second arrow is to the first one, regardless of whether either is near the target).

These same principles also apply to measurement (assessment) tools. A kitchen scale (weighing scale) can be used to illustrate the different concepts:
  • If the scale claims to measure weight and does so, then the scale is valid.
  • If it provides the same reading regardless of who uses it or when they use it, then the scale is reliable.
  • If the reading is correct when a known standard weight is weighed, then the scale is accurate.
  • If repeated weighings of the same item give the same reading (whether accurate or not), then the scale is precise.

they are stable over time.[69] However, it is because they are stable over time that they should not and cannot be used to detect change after an intervention.[70] Robust research is one of the backbones for improving clinical care for individuals with CP. The classification systems are very useful for research since participants can be better identified for research studies.

Finally, although CP is a single diagnosis, it is far from a uniform condition. Similar to autism, a name change, from "cerebral palsy" to "cerebral palsy spectrum disorder," has been suggested.[71]

When you have a child with GMFCS IV or V, it feels like every questionnaire or form you fill out at the doctor's or therapist's office focuses on everything your child cannot do. It gets very disheartening to fill out these forms, always answering the questions with, "No, my child still cannot do that." We are 14 years into these types of forms, and it still bothers me to this day. I just have to remind myself that although my child cannot do any of the tasks listed, he can still smile and spread joy and love, and he is perfect in his own way. I acknowledge the short pity party in my head and allow myself to briefly feel the frustration these forms bring. Then I move on and focus on the positive because it does no good to dwell on the things we cannot change.

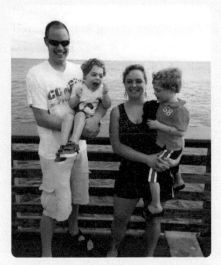

Chris holding Levi and Kate holding Cam.

The International Classification of Functioning, Disability and Health

The individual is rarely going to be altered very much, whereas the environment slowly but surely can.

Tom Shakespeare

The International Classification of Functioning, Disability and Health (ICF), a framework briefly addressed in the Introduction, is considered here in more detail and in the context of CP. The ICF was developed by WHO* in 2001 to help show the impact of a health condition at different levels and how those levels are interconnected. It tells us to look at the full picture—to look at the person with a disability in their life situation. The "F" in the short-form name of the framework (the ICF) stands for "functioning," which shows where its emphasis lies.

The framework provides a way of looking at the concepts of health and disability. It shows that every human being can experience a decrease in health and thereby experience some disability. That is, disability is

---

* When WHO (the World Health Organization) was established in 1948, it defined health as "… a state of complete physical, mental, and social well-being and not merely the absence of disease or infirmity." This interesting and broad definition has stood the test of time: it has never been amended.

not something that happens only to a minority of people. The ICF thus "mainstreams" disability and recognizes it as a widespread human experience. See Figure 1.8.1.

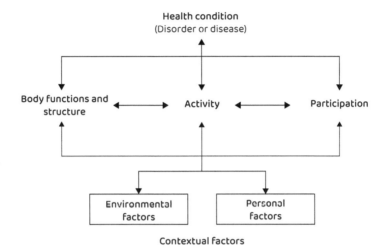

Figure 1.8.1 International Classification of Functioning, Disability and Health (ICF). Reproduced with kind permission from WHO.

The framework describes three levels of human functioning and disability as difficulty functioning at one or more of these three levels:[1]

- **Body functions and structure** refers to functioning at the level of the body or a body part.* For example, spasticity, muscle weakness, pain, and cognition are at this level. Impairments are defined as problems in body functions and structure.
- **Activity** is performing a task or action by an individual; for example, communicating or feeding. Activity limitations are difficulties an individual may have in performing activities.
- **Participation** is involvement in life situations. Playing sports with friends or attending school are examples. Participation restrictions are difficulties an individual may experience being involved in life situations.

---

* WHO formally defines "body functions" as physiological functions of body systems (including psychological functions). "Body structures" are defined as anatomical parts of the body such as organs, limbs, and their components.

The framework also includes factors that influence any of the three levels of functioning (termed "contextual factors"):

- **Environmental factors** make up the physical, social, and attitudinal environment in which people live. Examples include structural barriers at home and in the community, such as steps or stairs without handrails in the house, or a school with stairs but no elevator.
- **Personal factors** include gender, age, social background, education, past and present experiences, and other factors that influence how the person experiences disability. Examples include a person's attitude, determination, motivation, and resilience.

The three levels of human functioning, plus environmental and personal factors, are all interconnected with the health condition. The ICF shifts the focus from the *cause* to the *impact* of a health condition at the different levels.

Regarding activity, the ICF distinguishes between motor capacity and motor performance:

- **Motor capacity** is what a person can do in a standardized, controlled environment (e.g., a child at an appointment and walking on a smooth surface with the medical professional and parent watching and encouraging them).
- **Motor performance** is what a person actually does in their daily environment (e.g., a child walking in a crowded playground on uneven surfaces).

There is a third concept to keep in mind when considering activity: motor capability, which is what a person can do in their daily environment.[72] For example, a child may be able to ride a bike to school—they have the capability—but they may choose not to. Their performance is influenced by their choice. Physical and social environment and personal factors such as motivation influence the relationship between capacity, capability, and performance.[72]

A series of "F-words" has been developed and inserted into the different areas of the ICF, providing a useful adaptation of the framework (see Figure 1.8.2).[73] "Fitness," "functioning," "friends," "family," "fun," and "future" are highlighted as areas of focus for the child with a health condition. Indeed, these also apply to adults. A number of useful videos on the F-words are included in **Useful web resources.**

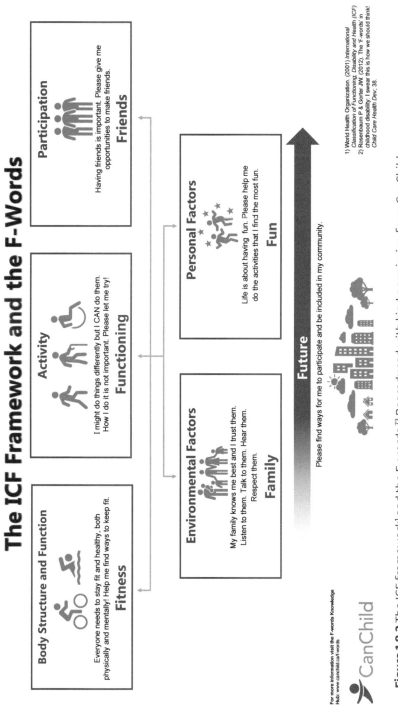

Figure 1.8.2 The ICF Framework[1] and the F-words.[73] Reproduced with kind permission from CanChild.

Key points Chapter 1

- CP is a group of conditions caused by an injury to the developing brain that can result in a variety of motor and other problems that affect how the child functions. Because the injury occurs in a developing brain and growing child, problems often change over time, even though the brain injury itself is unchanging.
- CP is a lifelong condition. There is currently no cure, nor is one imminent, but good management and treatment can help alleviate some or many of the effects of the brain injury.
- Seventy to 80 percent of CP cases are associated with prenatal factors, and birth asphyxia (insufficient oxygen during birth) plays a relatively minor role.
- Infants who are born preterm (earlier than 37 weeks) or who have low birth weight have a higher risk of CP.
- The current CP birth prevalence for high-income countries is declining and is now 1.6 per 1,000 live births. It is higher for low- and middle-income countries.
- The most recent report from the Australian Cerebral Palsy Register shows a decrease in both prevalence and severity of CP.
- Using certain standardized tests in combination with clinical examination and medical history, a diagnosis of CP can often accurately be made before six months corrected age.
- Confirmation of the presence of a brain injury by magnetic resonance imaging (MRI) occurs in many but not all individuals with CP. Up to 17 percent of children given the diagnosis of CP have normal MRI brain scans.
- Early diagnosis is very important because it allows for early intervention. Early intervention helps to achieve better functional outcomes for the child.
- CP can be classified based on the predominant motor type (the predominant abnormal muscle tone and movement impairment) and topography (area of the body affected).
- A number of classification systems describe the functional mobility (as in movement from place to place), manual ability (ability to handle objects), communication ability, eating and drinking ability, and visual function of individuals with CP.

Spastic quadriplegia

Introduction

You see things; and you say "Why?" But I dream
things that never were; and I say "Why not?"
George Bernard Shaw

This book addresses spastic quadriplegic CP GMFCS levels IV and V. This is a complex or severe form of CP. This chapter aims to contribute to understanding how the condition arises and develops over time. It provides much of the information that parents want to know early on as they consider the future for their newly diagnosed child. Every child with spastic quadriplegia GMFCS levels IV and V is unique and has their own individual strengths and challenges.

Receiving a diagnosis of spastic quadriplegia is difficult. Children with spastic quadriplegia are often medically complex, and their care can be challenging for both the family and themselves.

The complex care needs of children with spastic quadriplegia necessitate a multidisciplinary approach, as no single profession or discipline possesses the comprehensive expertise or range to address all aspects of their care.[74] The system of care delivery for these medically complex children is often termed the "medical home."[75] The medical home is a model for "providing accessible, family-centered, continuous, comprehensive, coordinated, compassionate, and culturally effective care to patients with the goal of improved health outcomes."[75]

Children with spastic quadriplegia are frequently born at term and may have an extensive brain injury.[3] Spastic quadriplegia involves the upper and the lower limbs and trunk; the degree of involvement often varies between the upper and the lower limbs and between the two sides of the body. The diagnosis of spastic quadriplegia is usually made early in life when the child is in a period of rapid growth. At that time, the child's joints are still flexible, but their affected muscles are already beginning to pull on their bones and joints in generally predictable patterns. This contributes to changes in posture and positioning that often can be manageable when the child is small but become more difficult as they grow. As growth continues, they may develop muscle contractures* and stiffness in their muscles and joints. Contractures occur when the muscles and tendons become tight and shortened causing flexing (bending) or stiffening of joints. This commonly occurs in the shoulders, elbows, wrists, hips, knees, and feet.

Individuals with spastic quadriplegia frequently have a distinct appearance due to muscle contractures and stiffness. Muscle contractures and stiffness can lead to functional limitations in performing daily activities, including mobility, dressing, grooming, and eating, and can often cause pain and discomfort. Some individuals with spastic quadriplegia may have difficulty smiling or frowning due to muscle and movement challenges in their face. In addition, some may have unwanted movements.

Distribution across classification systems

In Chapter 1, we saw how CP could be classified using a number of classification systems including functional mobility (GMFCS), ability to handle objects (MACS), communication ability (CFCS), eating and drinking ability (EDACS), and visual function (VFCS). Figure 2.1.1 summarizes the percentage of children with spastic quadriplegia across

---

* A muscle contracture is a limitation of a joint's range of motion (ROM).[76] The terms "muscle contracture" and "tight muscle" are used interchangeably in the CP field and in this book.

the five levels of the GMFCS and MACS.[45,77,78,79] No studies were found that separately identified children with spastic quadriplegia across the five levels of the CFCS, EDACS, and VFCS, but in general, though not always, they are at higher levels for those classification systems also.

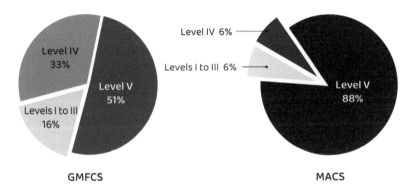

Figure 2.1.1 Distribution of children with spastic quadriplegia across the GMFCS[45,77,78,79] and MACS.[78]

Figure 2.1.1 shows that for children with spastic quadriplegia, 84 percent were at levels IV and V for functional mobility (GMFCS) and 94 percent were at levels IV and V for ability to handle objects (MACS).

This book is relevant to those at GMFCS levels IV and V, which account for the majority of individuals with spastic quadriplegia.

Co-occurring motor type

In Chapter 1, we saw that CP can be classified based on the predominant motor type, which in the case of spastic quadriplegia is spasticity. Individuals with spastic quadriplegia often have secondary, or co-occurring, motor types, hence the term "mixed movement disorder." Data from the Australian CP register shows that 48 percent of individuals with spastic quadriplegia have co-occurring dyskinesia, while 3 percent have co-occurring hypotonia.[*42] It is believed that the true prevalence of co-occurring motor types is higher.[4] A more recent study found that 50 percent of children and young people with CP (all types) had spasticity and dystonia. The presence of dystonia with spasticity

* For those who acquired CP in the prenatal or perinatal period only; also includes triplegia.

has been underrecognized.[48] This is important because the management of spasticity and dystonia is different.

Associated problems

A large Australian study reported the prevalence of associated problems among children age five with spastic quadriplegia across all GMFCS levels.[80] See Figure 2.1.2.

	No problems	Mild/Some	Severe problems
Speech	No problems 11%	Some problems 28%	Approximately 3 in 5 are nonverbal 61%
Intelligence	No or probably no problems 26%	Mild/probable problems 32%	Approximately 2 in 5 have moderate to severe intellectual problems 42%
Vision	Almost 1 in 2 have no problems 45%	Some problems 39%	Functionally blind 16%
Epilepsy	None 43%	Resolved by age 5 5%	Approximately 1 in 2 have epilepsy 53%
Hearing	Approximately 4 in 5 have no problems 82%	Some problems 13%	Bilateral deafness 5%

Figure 2.1.2 Prevalence of associated problems among children age five with spastic quadriplegia (all GMFCS levels). Data also includes children with triplegia.

Figure 2.1.2 shows that almost all children age five with spastic quadriplegia have problems with speech, and three in five are nonverbal. Three-quarters of children have some level of intellectual problems. More than half have some level of vision problems, and more than half have epilepsy. However, hearing is unaffected in many. Not shown in the figure is that half the children have two or more severe associated problems.[80] The prevalence and severity of associated problems were found to be greater in children at higher GMFCS levels compared with those at lower GMFCS levels.[80]

In this chapter, we address the brain injury and explain how it affects the development of the musculoskeletal problems. However, spastic quadriplegia affects many more body systems, and its effects may reduce well-being far more than the musculoskeletal problems. The effects of spastic quadriplegia across other body systems is addressed in Chapter 3.

Finally, where possible, the research studies cited here are relevant to those with spastic quadriplegia GMFCS levels IV and V. In those studies that include multiple subtypes, we aim to indicate the proportion of individuals with spastic quadriplegia and/or GMFCS level. Where data was available only for bilateral CP, we have included that. Sometimes, information about CP in general is included, where it is useful.

USEFUL WEB RESOURCES

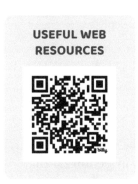

What does best practice look like?

Medicine is a science of uncertainty and an art of probability.
Sir William Osler

It is important to understand what best practice in the medical care of individuals with spastic quadriplegia looks like. We saw in section 2.1 that the medical home is a model for "providing accessible, family-centered, continuous, comprehensive, coordinated, compassionate, and culturally effective care to patients with the goal of improved health outcomes."[75] The complex care needs of children with spastic quadriplegia necessitate a multidisciplinary approach, as no single profession or discipline possesses the comprehensive expertise or range to address all aspects of their care.[74] This section provides an overview of the generally accepted principles underpinning best practice in the management and treatment of spastic quadriplegia at the time of writing. Best practice is likely to continue to evolve over time. It currently includes:

- Family-centered care and person-centered care
- A multidisciplinary team approach
- Evidence-based medicine and shared decision-making
- Data-driven decision-making

- The importance of specialist centers
- Early intervention
- Setting goals
- Using measurement tools and measuring outcome

Family-centered care and person-centered care

When a child is diagnosed with spastic quadriplegia, the whole family is affected: parents, siblings, and extended family members. Family-centered care is a way of ensuring that care is planned around the whole family, not just the child with the condition.[*] It can be thought of as a meeting of experts who pool their knowledge to jointly develop the most appropriate plan of care for the child. The parent is the expert on their child, while the professional is the expert on the condition and its treatment. Professionals who practice family-centered care see themselves not as the sole authority but as a partner with the parent in the provision of care for the child.

Family-centered care and person-centered care are closely related. The latter evolves from the former as the child grows. In person-centered care, insofar as cognitive capacity allows, the individual is an active participant and decision maker in their own medical care. The change from family-centered care to person-centered care is gradual, and parents and medical professionals can help facilitate the shift over time.

A multidisciplinary team approach

A multidisciplinary team approach means the individual is being treated by medical professionals from several disciplines working together as a team, although each stays within their own professional boundaries. Optimal treatment for individuals with CP may include medical professionals from many disciplines, including physical therapy (PT);

---

[*] Family-centered care is also termed "family-centered service." CanChild defines family-centered care as being "made up of a set of values, attitudes, and approaches to services for children with special needs and their families. Family-centred service recognizes that **each family is unique**; that the family is the **constant in the child's life**; and that they are the **experts on the child's abilities and needs**. The family works with service providers to make informed decisions about the services and supports the child and family receive. In family-centred service, the strengths and needs of all family members are considered."[81]

occupational therapy (OT); speech and language pathology (SLP), also termed "speech and language therapy" (SLT); nursing; orthotics; pediatrics; neurology; neurosurgery; ophthalmology; orthopedic surgery; otolaryngology; pulmonology; gastroenterology; physical medicine and rehabilitation (PM&R), also termed "physiatry"; and more.*

A more detailed explanation of the role of the team members is included in Cerebral Palsy Road Map: What to Expect as Your Child Grows[82] (included in **Useful web resources**).

Evidence-based medicine and shared decision-making

Evidence-based medicine (or evidence-based practice) is "the conscientious, explicit, and judicious use of current best evidence in making decisions about the care of individual patients."[83] It combines the best available external clinical evidence from research with the clinical expertise of the professional.[83] Family priorities and preferences are also considered.[84] Since clinical expertise can vary, it is important to know that recommendations made in this book may be different at other hospitals and treatment centers.

Best practice management of CP is by a multidisciplinary team that is skilled in this condition and that engages with the family in a shared decision-making model. Shared decision-making is a process in which the family is actively involved in making the medical decisions. It incorporates the principles of evidence-based medicine.[85]

---

* The role of PT, OT, and SLP is explained in section 4.2. **Gastroenterology** deals with disorders of the digestive system, including the stomach and intestines. **Neurology** deals with disorders of the nervous system. **Neurosurgery** involves surgical management of disorders of the nervous system. **Orthotics** is concerned with the design, manufacture, and management of orthoses, devices designed to hold specific body parts in position to modify their structure and/or function. **Ophthalmology** deals with disorders of vision and eye health concerns. **Orthopedic surgery** involves surgical management of disorders affecting the musculoskeletal system: the muscles, bones, joints, and their related structures. **Otolaryngology** deals with disorders of ear, nose, and throat (also termed "ear, nose, and throat" or ENT). Pediatrics deals with children and their medical conditions. **PM&R** aims to enhance and restore functional ability and quality of life among those with physical disabilities. **Pulmonology** deals with disorders of the respiratory system, particularly the lungs and airway.

Unfortunately, though evidence-based practice is the goal, several authors in the field of CP have noted that there is a long way to go to achieve it.[86,87] The translation of research into clinical practice can be slow: this applies to all medical fields, not just CP. It has been found that it takes an average of 17 years for research evidence to reach clinical practice.[88] For example, the GMFCS was first published in 1997, but a 2015 published survey of 283 pediatric physical therapists found that fewer than half used the GMFCS consistently,[89] and a 2018 study found that fewer than half of 303 caregivers knew their child's GMFCS level.[90]

Implementation science is an emerging field of health care science that focuses on bridging the gap between research and its effective implementation in clinical practice. Factors that influence successful implementation include organizational behavior, clinician behavior, and patient preference. An example is the successful implementation of the guideline for early detection of CP across a network of five US high-risk infant follow-up programs.[24] Another is the development and rollout of COVID-19 vaccines.

Funding for CP research is low, which makes the choice of research conducted very important. A 2018 US initiative to set a person-centered research agenda for CP involved a collaboration of all stakeholders—including caregivers and people with CP—based on the belief that a research agenda developed collaboratively would be more useful to the entire community than one developed by professionals alone. It was built around the concept of "nothing about us without us."*[91]

Finally, given that research is the cornerstone of advancing medical science, it is worth noting that a simple search in PubMed† of "cerebral palsy GMFCS level X" across the five GMFCS levels revealed 1,145 results for GMFCS level I and six results for GMFCS level V. This difference does not reflect the relative number of individuals across GMFCS levels. The fact that more severe forms of CP are less represented in research studies needs to be addressed.

---

* Sixteen top research priorities were identified. Leading themes included the comparative effectiveness of interventions, physical activity, and understanding aging. It also highlighted the need to focus on longitudinal research that includes outcomes related to participation and quality of life.

† A free online database of medical and life sciences research articles.

Data-driven decision-making

Best practice demands decision-making be data-driven. (This can also be called "data-informed decision-making.") For example, in orthopedic surgical decision-making in spastic quadriplegia, data is drawn from multiple sources, including:

- The individual's history
- Functional outcome measures and family-reported outcome measures
- Physical examination
- Imaging

The skilled evaluation of multiple sources of data is essential for good decision-making.

The importance of specialist centers

Specialist centers, or centers of excellence, are on the rise in many areas of medicine across the developed world. Consider, for example, specialist centers for breast cancer. Research has shown that outcomes in breast cancer treatment improve with the number of breast cancer cases a particular center has treated (this is known as centralization).[92] The annual number of operations per center and per surgeon (specialization) is also important, and the multidisciplinary team is paramount.[92]

A specialist center for the treatment of individuals with CP:

- Has a multidisciplinary team that includes the specialties described earlier
- Treats a high volume of patients with CP on a routine or daily basis
- Provides the full range of evidence-based treatment options, allowing the most suitable ones to be chosen for each child
- Conducts research and publishes in peer-reviewed journals
- Ideally, offers a lifetime of care; CP is not just a "children's condition"

Early intervention

Early intervention is essential in the management of CP. Early intervention is usually from birth to age three in the US[93] and may continue beyond that age elsewhere. We have already seen that:

- Early diagnosis is necessary for early intervention.
- Early intervention offers the best opportunity to tap into neuroplasticity.
- Early intervention is important for minimizing the secondary problems as the child grows. Remember, growth is most vigorous in the first three years of life.

In addition to helping train parents in how to care for and best help their child learn, early intervention can help with adaptations to make the home environment more conducive to learning. Early intervention can also help with access to assistive technology for mobility, communication, and vision, which helps to maximize the child's ability to interact, participate, and learn.

Though the emphasis with intervention is on early implementation, intervention continues to be required during childhood, adolescence, and adulthood.

Setting goals

Treatment goals should be collaboratively agreed upon by the family and professional as part of family-centered care and shared decision-making. The achievement of goals should be evaluated after treatment. One widely used goal-directed system used in rehabilitation is known as SMART, a system applied in many industries in areas like project management and employee performance. It is also used in personal development.

The SMART system goals are designed to be Specific, Measurable, Achievable, Relevant, and Time-bound:[94]

- **Specific** and **Measurable:** Goals that are specific and measurable should contain five elements:

- o Who
- o Will do what
- o Under what conditions
- o How well
- o By when
- **Achievable:** Goals should match the child's prognosis and be attainable.
- **Relevant:** Goals should hold meaning for the child and family. Goals should be functional; that is, not solely based on impairment (problems with body functions and structure).
- **Time-bound:** Goals must have a specific date for achievement.

The following are some examples of SMART goals:

- Kelly will use both hands to hold a toy for one minute when supported in sitting within one month.[*]
- Cosmas will bring hand to mouth to participate in self-feeding while positioned in chair within one month.
- Cadence will "army crawl" (crawl on belly) 10 feet (3 meters) to access toys in playroom within six weeks.
- Anna will stand upright in stander for 10 minutes to interact at eye level with her sibling within one month.
- Amelia will drive her power wheelchair safely from room to room within her home within one month.
- Simon will initiate requests for a preferred activity 80 percent of given opportunities using total communication (i.e., speech, signs, pointing and/or using his Touch Talker) within one month.

Research has shown that:

- Therapies that focus on achieving functional goals in everyday life result in measurable improvements in gross motor skills compared to therapies that are not goal-directed.[95]
- The development of fewer and more meaningful goals is imperative for adherence, improved outcomes, and greater individual and family satisfaction.[96]

---

[*] Typically, a goal would include a specific date for achievement, rather than the less specific "within one month."

- A family-centered approach to intervention has been shown to improve motivation and outcome.[97]

A number of tools are available to incorporate family goals. Some of the more common ones are the Canadian Occupational Performance Measure (COPM),[98] the Goal Attainment Scale,[99] and the Gait Outcomes Assessment List (GOAL).[100–103]

Using measurement tools and measuring outcome

Many variables can be measured, including height, weight, and functional ability. Some variables can be measured using equipment, and others by parent or self-report (e.g., by completing a questionnaire). A tape measure, a scale, and CPCHILD (see below) are all examples of tools used to measure variables. A measurement can be taken at any time to establish a person's status at that point in time.

An outcome is defined as a result or an effect; thus, "measuring outcome" means measuring a result or an effect. If a person's weight is measured before a treatment such as a change in feeding regimen and then again afterward, one can evaluate the effect or result—the outcome—of the new feeding regimen on the person's weight by comparing the before and after measurements. The outcome of the new feeding regimen can thus be measured using the variable of weight. Many types of measurement tools are used to assess outcome.

Variables used to measure outcome can be classified as technical (e.g., weight), functional (e.g., ability to self-feed), or patient/parent satisfaction (e.g., family satisfaction with new feeding regimen). Each variable provides different but complementary information. Variables can be measured in each domain of the ICF (body functions and structure, activity, and participation). A range of variables (technical, functional, and patient/parent satisfaction) covering different domains of the ICF provides the most comprehensive evaluation of outcome.

CPCHILD is a measurement tool specifically developed for children with severe developmental disabilities.[104] It comprises 37 questions (items) and measures caregiver's perspectives across six areas:

- Personal care/activities of daily living
- Positioning, transferring, and mobility
- Comfort and emotions
- Communication and social interaction
- Health
- Overall quality of life

It can also measure the importance of each item on the child's quality of life. It is very useful to measure outcome after an intervention; for example, scoliosis surgery. More information is included in **Useful web resources.**

Common measurement tools may need to be adapted for individuals with spastic quadriplegia by incorporating alternative formats, such as simplified language, visual aids, or physical accommodations, to ensure accurate evaluation of abilities.

Overall management philosophy

When there is no turning back, then we should concern ourselves only with the best way of going forward.

Paulo Coelho

For the child and adolescent with spastic quadriplegia, the management of all aspects of the condition can be a full-time job for parents. Some children and adolescents with spastic quadriplegia are generally quite healthy while others have many challenges. There is, as a matter of necessity, a way to prioritize management—it begins with assuring general health before addressing participation. For example, if a person is struggling with chronic respiratory or stomach issues, they do not have the energy to put toward other tasks such as development, play, or learning. This is true for all of us. Our general health is the foundation that allows us to participate in life. Therefore, this section lays out care priorities and an overall management philosophy for children and adolescents with spastic quadriplegia. And while we address management under different headings, it is crucial to bear in mind that the body operates as a unified entity, and body systems are intricately interlinked and interdependent.

Level 1 considerations, general health, are addressed in Chapter 3:

- Respiratory system
- Feeding, swallowing, and nutrition
- Digestive system
- Urinary system
- Epilepsy
- Sleep
- Pain
- Sensory system

Level 2 considerations, developmental progress and maximizing function, are addressed in Chapter 4:

- Therapies
- The home program
- Assistive technology

Level 3 considerations, musculoskeletal health—orthopedic care, are addressed in Chapter 5:

- Tone reduction
- Musculoskeletal surveillance
- Orthopedic surgery

Level 4 considerations, increasing participation, are addressed in Chapter 6:

- Cognition and intelligence
- Mental and behavioral health
- Puberty and sexual expression
- Community integration

Chapter 7 addresses alternative and complementary treatments. Chapter 8 addresses the transition to adulthood, which is then addressed in Chapter 9.

For those who would like more background reading, an explanation of the development of function is included in **Useful web resources.**

However, before we address management of spastic quadriplegia in Chapters 3 to 9, we first explain the brain injury and the musculoskeletal problems associated with the condition.

The brain injury

Do not let what you cannot do interfere with what you can do.

John Wooden

The effects and severity of brain injury that causes CP depend on when (timing in development) and where (location in the brain) it occurs, and that translates to the subtype of CP. Different subtypes result from injury at different times in development and to different areas of the brain. The brain injury of spastic quadriplegia is extensive and involves both sides of the brain and all four limbs and trunk.

A Canadian study reported the most common causes of spastic quadriplegia as perinatal hypoxic ischemic encephalopathy (HIE) (33 percent), periventricular leukomalacia (15 percent), central nervous system infections (11 percent), other (23 percent), and unknown (17 percent).[105]

Hypoxic ischemic encephalopathy (HIE) is a condition where the brain doesn't receive enough oxygen and bloodflow, causing brain injury. The following explains the terms:

- "Hypoxic" from "hypoxia" means a reduction in the amount of oxygen reaching the tissue.
- "Ischemic" from "ischemia" means an inadequate amount of blood to a part of the body.
- "Encephalopathy" means any injury to the brain that alters brain function or structure.

Periventricular leukomalacia (PVL) is a brain injury characterized by damage to the white matter surrounding the brain's ventricles.* The following explains the terms:

- "Periventricular" means "around the ventricles." The injury occurs *near* ("peri") these ventricles.
- "Leuko" means "white" and "malacia" means "abnormal softening of tissue." The term "leukomalacia," therefore, means "softening of the white tissue."

The full term, "periventricular leukomalacia," thus means, "softening of the white tissue around the ventricles."

Central nervous system infections include meningitis (the inflammation of the membranes, or meninges, surrounding the brain) and encephalitis (inflammation of the brain tissue itself).[105]

Other causes include:[105]

- Malformation (abnormal development of brain structures)
- Metabolic diseases (disruption in biochemical processes affecting brain development and/or function)
- Genetic cause (inherited conditions or mutations affecting brain development and/or function)
- Intraventricular hemorrhage (bleeding inside the brain's ventricles)
- Hydrocephalus (accumulation of cerebrospinal fluid in the brain)
- Kernicterus (a brain injury resulting from untreated jaundice)
- Vascular cause (disruption in blood supply to the brain)

---

* The ventricles are interconnected fluid-filled cavities that produce, circulate, and contain cerebrospinal fluid, which protects the brain and spinal cord.

Musculoskeletal system

Strength does not come from physical capacity.
It comes from an indomitable will.

Mahatma Gandhi

The child with spastic quadriplegia is born with what appear to be typical muscles, bones, and joints, but over time the typical physical features of spastic quadriplegia GMFCS levels IV and V develop as they grow. (See Table 2.5.1.) Individuals with spastic quadriplegia can have some, but not necessarily all, these features.

Table 2.5.1 Typical physical features of spastic quadriplegia GMFCS levels IV and V

TERM	EXPLANATION	ILLUSTRATION
Spine		
Scoliosis	A three-dimensional rotation and curvature of the spine. The spine on the left in the image is typical, the spine on the right has scoliosis	
Shoulder and upper limb		
Adducted shoulder	The arm is moved inward toward the middle of the body (midline).	
Inwardly rotated shoulder	The upper arm is turned internally toward the body.	
Flexed elbow	The arm is bent at the elbow. It is difficult to extend and straighten the elbow.	
Pronated forearm	The hand is in the palm down position.	
Flexed wrist	The wrist is bent downward. It is difficult to extend and straighten the wrist.	

Cont'd.

TERM	EXPLANATION	ILLUSTRATION
Shoulder and upper limb		
Adducted and flexed thumb	The thumb is bent and positioned toward the middle finger. This is also termed "thumb in palm."	
Flexed fingers	The fingers are folded in toward the palm. This is the clenched fist and curled thumb so often seen in spastic quadriplegia.	
Lower limb		
Hip displacement (subluxation, dislocation)	Hip displacement: the degree to which the head (ball) of the femur (thigh bone) is out of the acetabulum (socket) of the hip bone: • Hip subluxation: the ball is partially out of the socket but is still in contact with it; it is still partially covered by the socket. • Hip dislocation: the ball is completely out of the socket. The subject's right hip in the image is normal, while their left hip is dislocated.	
Windswept hips	The subject's right hip in the image is in adduction and internal rotation, while their left hip is in abduction and external rotation.*	
Flexion at the hips and knees	The hips and knees are bent.	

* Hip adduction is movement of the thigh toward the midline. Hip internal rotation is rotary movement of the thigh toward the midline. Hip abduction is movement of the thigh away from the midline. Hip external rotation is rotary movement of the thigh away from the midline.

Cont'd.

TERM	EXPLANATION	ILLUSTRATION
Lower limb		
Genu valgus	The femurs (thigh bones) turn inward, causing the knees to touch while the ankles remain apart. This is commonly referred to as "knock knees."	
Equinus	The feet are pointed downward.	
Talipes equinovarus (TEV) or, simply, equinovarus	The foot is pointed downward (equino) and inward (varus). In addition, the arch is increased, and the heel is turned inward. This is commonly referred to as clubfoot.	
Equinovalgus	The foot is pointed downward (equino) and the heel pointed outward (valgus).	
Planovalgus	The arch of the foot is flat (plano) and the heel pointed outward (valgus).	
Hallux valgus	A bony protrusion on the inner edge of the left foot. It appears as if the big toe is bending toward the other four toes. Also called a bunion.	

For those who would like more background reading, a detailed explanation of bones, joints, muscles, and movements is included in Appendix 2 (online).

The motor system or neuromusculoskeletal system involves the nervous system, muscles, bones, and their related structures. Based on clinical expertise, Gage proposed a useful framework for classifying the neuromusculoskeletal problems that occur in children with spastic CP.[106,107] Problems are categorized as primary, secondary, and tertiary:

- Primary problems are caused by the brain injury and are therefore present from when the brain injury occurred. Many are neurological problems but may also include alterations in the structure of the muscles themselves.
- Secondary problems develop over time in the growing child. They are problems of atypical muscle growth and bone development and are referred to as "growth problems."
- Tertiary problems are the "coping responses" that arise to compensate for or counteract the primary and secondary problems.

We now address:

- **Growth**
- **Primary problems**
- **Secondary problems**
- **Tertiary problems**

Growth

The musculoskeletal problems in spastic quadriplegia develop in proportion to growth; therefore, an understanding of growth is helpful. Growth occurs in three major phases during a child's life: birth to age three, three years to puberty, and puberty to maturity. Of the three, two are of *rapid* growth: from birth to three years and during puberty.[108] The rate of growth that occurs in these two phases is particularly important for the child with spastic quadriplegia because musculoskeletal problems emerge with growth.

A large US study of growth in children and adolescents with CP led to the development of growth charts for boys and girls with CP age 2 to 20. These were developed for each GMFCS level.[109,110] The study found that children and adolescents with CP (all subtypes) are shorter than typically developing peers (Figures 2.5.1 and 2.5.2). It also found that boys and girls at GMFCS level V who are tube-fed (liquid nutrition delivered through a plastic tube placed in the stomach or small intestine) grow better than those who feed orally (food and drink taken by mouth). Feeding is addressed in Chapter 3.

These growth charts are included in **Useful web resources.**

Similar trends in height difference among children and adolescents with CP have been observed in other parts of the world.[111]

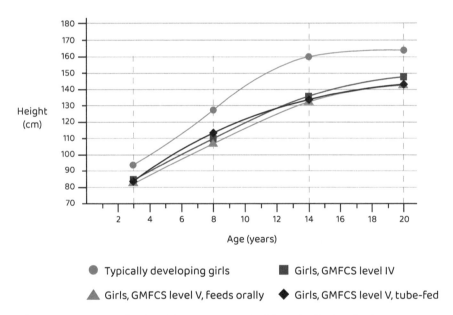

Figure 2.5.1 Height of girls with CP compared with typically developing peers. Data shows the 50th percentile height at various ages. Data collated and compiled from references.[109,110,112,113]

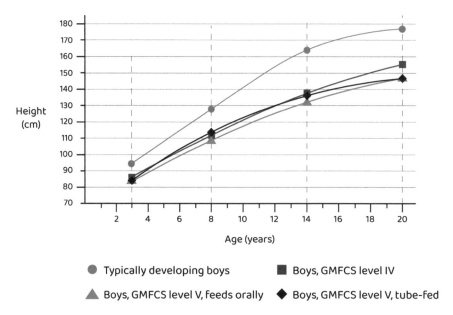

Figure 2.5.2 Height of boys with CP compared with typically developing peers. Data shows the 50th percentile height at various ages. Data collated and compiled from references.[109,110,114,115]

Primary problems

As we saw above, primary problems are caused by the brain injury and are therefore present from when the brain injury occurred. Primary problems include the following, and each is examined in turn:

- Lack of selective motor control
- Poor balance
- Abnormal tone
- Muscle weakness
- Sensory problems

Even though the above items are listed separately, it does not mean they manifest independently; nor does it mean they equally impact the various outcomes or concerns of individuals with CP.

a) Lack of selective motor control

In simple terms, selective motor control refers to the ability to isolate a muscle or combination of muscles to produce a particular movement. Lack of selective motor control results from the brain injury and the disruption of messages from the cerebrum and other areas of the brain.

b) Poor balance

In the context of the body, balance is the ability to maintain stability and equilibrium while stationary or in motion. Adequate balance is important, for example, in maintaining head and trunk control, and the task of maintaining balance for sitting independently can be complex. Sitting involves head and body righting, but it also involves adjustments to the body's positioning relative to other stimuli in the environment (e.g., hitting a bump on the road while riding in a wheelchair). Balance is one of the areas affected in spastic quadriplegia as a result of the brain injury.

c) Abnormal tone

Muscle tone is the resting tension in a muscle. A range of "normal" muscle tone exists. Tone is considered "abnormal" when it falls outside the range of normal or typical. It can be too low (hypotonia) or too high (hypertonia). Abnormal muscle tone occurs in all types of CP. In children with spastic quadriplegia, tone is typically too high in the legs and arms, but it can be low in the trunk.

i) Spasticity

Spasticity is one type of high tone. There are a number of definitions of spasticity. One is that it is a condition in which there is an abnormal increase in muscle tone or stiffness of muscle that can interfere with movement and speech, and be associated with discomfort or pain.[22] Another definition highlights the velocity-dependent nature of spasticity.[116]

A muscle reacts to rapid stretching by contracting in opposition (i.e., the muscle tightens rather than continuing to stretch or lengthen). This is designed to protect the muscle from overstretching when quickly stretched. See Figure 2.5.3.

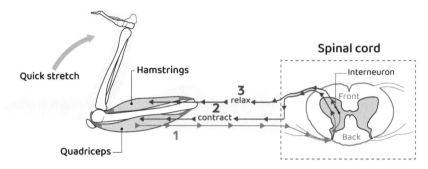

Figure 2.5.3 Example of a "normal" stretch reflex. **1.** Quadriceps are stretched quickly, and information is sent via sensory neurons to the spinal cord. **2.** Motor neurons cause the quadriceps to contract to resist the quick stretch. **3.** Motor neurons cause the hamstrings to relax to allow the quadriceps to contract.

- A **"normal" stretch reflex** is a rapid, involuntary muscle contraction (in quadriceps shown in Figure 2.5.3) in response to a sudden stretch of the muscle.*
- A **"hyperactive" stretch reflex** is an exaggerated reflex response that leads to excessive muscle contraction and increased muscle tone. Spasticity is a hyperactive stretch reflex (the excessive muscle contraction can be felt as resistance by a person doing a quick passive stretch of the muscle).†

The speed of the rapid stretch is important because the spastic reaction happens only with a *quick* stretch. If the stretch is slow, it does not elicit a spastic reaction. (The effect of speed can be noted by comparing a muscle's response to slow versus quick passive stretching.)

Spasticity results from a loss of inhibition—the dampening input from specific nerve cells in the brain to nerve cells in the spinal cord, and hence to certain muscles.

Clonus is the most extreme form of spasticity, defined as a series of involuntary, rhythmic muscular contractions and relaxations. It can be seen in the gastrocnemius (one of the calf muscles); for example, when an examiner quickly dorsiflexes the foot (moves the foot up), the foot may then plantar flex (move down) and continue to move up and

---

* Doctors routinely perform a knee-jerk reflex test using a small rubber hammer to check for healthy reflex responses.

† Passive stretching is when another person stretches an individual's muscle.

down uncontrollably for a number of beats (contraction and relaxation cycles). A video depicting clonus is included in **Useful web resources.**

ii) Dyskinesia

Data from the Australian CP register shows that 48 percent of individuals with spastic quadriplegia* have co-occurring dyskinesia.[42] Dyskinesia is subdivided into dystonia and choreo-athetosis:[38]

- **Dystonia** is involuntary (unintended) muscle contractions that cause slow repetitive movements or abnormal postures. They can sometimes be painful.[39] Some define dystonia as muscles that "contract that you do not want to contract when you try to move." In contrast to spasticity, dystonia does not occur as a result of rapid stretch. Examples of dystonia include the leg muscles tightening or uncontrolled posturing movements of the fingers or toes when surprised, talking, or playing a video game (where there is excitement or tension).
- **Choreo-athetosis** includes features of both chorea and athetosis. Chorea is characterized by jerky, dance-like movements.[3] Athetosis is characterized by slow, writhing movements.[3] Thus, individuals with choreo-athetotic CP experience a combination of both choreic and athetoid movements. The main cause of choreo-athetosis is kernicterus (a brain injury), which is due to untreated jaundice in infancy. As a result of advances in health care, kernicterus has disappeared in many areas of developed countries; there, dystonia accounts for the majority of dyskinesia. However, kernicterus remains a problem in developing countries and in some rural, remote, or socioeconomically disadvantaged areas in developed countries.

A recent study found that 50 percent of Australian children and young people with CP (all types) had spasticity *and* dystonia.[48] The authors concluded that the presence of dystonia with spasticity has been under-recognized.[48] This is important because the management of spasticity and dystonia is different.

---

* For those who acquired CP in the prenatal or perinatal period only; also includes triplegia.

iii) Hypotonia

Data from the Australian CP register shows that three percent of individuals with spastic quadriplegia have co-occurring hypotonia.[42] Hypotonia is an abnormal decrease in muscle tone.[22]

iv) Measuring abnormal muscle tone

Abnormal muscle tone can be measured using different measurement tools. See Table 2.5.2.

Table 2.5.2 Common measurement tools for abnormal muscle tone

MEASUREMENT TOOL	TYPE OF ABNORMAL MUSCLE TONE
Modified Ashworth Scale (MAS)[117,118]	Spasticity
Modified Tardieu Scale (MTS)[118,119]	Spasticity
Barry-Albright Dystonia Scale (BADS)[120]	Dystonia
Hypertonia Assessment Tool (HAT)[121,122]	Dystonia and spasticity (and rigidity*).

* Rigidity is another type of high tone in which the muscles have the same amount of stiffness irrespective of the degree of movement. It is uncommon and practically does not exist in CP.

d) Muscle weakness

In general terms, muscle weakness is the inability to generate muscle force. Muscle strength can be measured by manual muscle testing or with a handheld machine called a dynamometer. Measuring muscle strength for people with CP is challenging because of the lack of selective motor control and contractures.

e) Sensory problems

"Sensory" refers to the senses. Sensory problems can include problems with vision and processing visual input, hearing and processing auditory input as well as decreased sensation, and a lack of awareness of the position and movement of the body (proprioception). Sensory problems are addressed in section 3.9.

The primary problems listed above are present from when the brain injury occurred. In general, the primary problems are difficult to change or improve. However, with diligent management, the impact of these primary problems can be minimized and function can be maximized.

Finally, even though primary problems are discussed separately, the problems exist together and they trend in similar directions (the level of effect of one is mirrored in others plus they can exacerbate one another). Primary problems should be evaluated and considered separately while recognizing that they may trend together. In general, the severity of primary problems is a significant predictor of GMFCS level.

Secondary problems

The secondary problems in spastic quadriplegia develop slowly over time and in direct proportion to the rate of bone growth. They also depend on the amount and type of usage of the muscles. We saw earlier that the periods of most rapid growth are from birth to age three and during puberty. These are, therefore, periods of great challenge and change in the child with spastic quadriplegia.

Secondary problems arise as a result of the atypical forces imposed on the growing skeleton by the effects of the primary brain injury and movement. In other words, the primary problems drive the secondary problems. Though secondary problems can be *somewhat* addressed by orthopedic surgery, surgery is a big undertaking for children and adolescents with spastic quadriplegia GMFCS levels IV and V as their general health status is often difficult to maintain.

This section covers:

- **Atypical muscle growth**
- **Atypical bone development**
- **Common muscle and bone problems in spastic quadriplegia**

a) Atypical muscle growth

What follows is a simplified explanation of atypical muscle growth in spastic quadriplegia. This is a very complex subject, and more is still being learned about the differences between muscles in typically developing individuals and in people with spastic CP. A muscle grows in length in response to stretch. It has been shown that for normal muscle lengthening to occur, two to four hours of stretching per day is required.[107] Bones grow during sleep,[123] and in a typically developing child, this required amount of stretching occurs when the child gets up and starts to move about, to run, and to play. This typical movement moves the joints and results in normal stretching of the muscles which provides the stimulus for laying down new muscle cells and is how a muscle grows in length. Thus, bone growth leads to stretching of the muscle, which leads to the muscle growing in length.

Because the primary problems predominantly affect the neuromusculoskeletal systems in children with spastic quadriplegia, they usually have decreased physical activity levels compared to typically developing children.[124] The reduced amount of physical activity can then affect their capacity to actively stretch their muscles. Even with movement, the child with spastic quadriplegia may not fully stretch out their muscles through the typical ROM of the joints. Thus, the reduced stretching range for many muscles may become the norm.

As a result, the muscles fail to grow adequately in length and width* and contractures develop,† which result in joints having reduced ROM. Indeed, in the past, CP was called "short muscle disease," although it's worth noting that, despite this title, the problem arises from muscles failing to grow in length and width rather than from becoming shortened. With lack of movement, the muscles also become stiff.

For young children with spastic quadriplegia, their muscles may still achieve their full ROM when they are relaxed; for example, during sleep. Over time, however, they may develop contracture, meaning that the full joint ROM cannot be achieved at any time. One study found decreasing ROM in the lower limb muscles in children with CP from age 2 to 14.[126]

Contractures interfere with positioning, movement, and function. For example, an elbow flexion contracture may result in limited ability to

---

* Muscles also grow in width. Growth in width has been shown to be decreased as well in children with CP.[125]

† More precisely, the contracture occurs in the muscle-tendon unit (MTU) and/or capsule of the joint, not just the muscle.

extend the elbow in reaching and make it difficult to perform activities such as dressing. Contractures may also interfere with the typical movements that lead to achieving gross motor milestones. Decreased mobility at any age may lead to activity limitation and reduced participation. Nordmark and colleagues described the circular nature of the problem: a decrease in ROM with age may result in decreased mobility, which in turn results in a further decrease in ROM—a vicious circle.[126]

In addition to the factors outlined above that may cause contractures to develop over time, there may be differences at a tissue level between muscles of individuals with CP and those of the typical population. These differences include: [3,125,127,128,129]

- **Smaller muscles** in both diameter and length, which may partially explain muscle weakness
- **Lengthened and fewer sarcomeres** (the functional unit of contraction of a muscle), though the muscle itself is shortened, this could also contribute to muscle weakness
- **Muscles being stiffer,** which is believed to be caused by atypical extracellular matrix (the network surrounding the muscle cells, consisting of collagen, proteins, and more)
- **Decrease in the number of satellite cells,** which are responsible for the majority of muscle growth
- **Increased fat and collagen,** which could contribute to muscle weakness even if the muscle is the same size

In summary, muscle quality and size may be different. Muscles may become smaller (less muscle bulk) and stiffer (less elastic) compared with those of typically developing children. Smaller muscle size has been reported in children with spastic CP compared to typically developing children and in children as young as 15 months.[130,131] It is to be expected that the muscles of a 14-year-old with spastic CP are very different from those of a 1-year-old with spastic CP. There is still more to learn about altered muscle composition in spastic CP.

To compensate for atypical muscle growth in a child with CP, parents have to ensure that their child gets adequate opportunity to stretch and move their spastic muscles. Traditionally, this included the parent doing daily slow stretches of the child's spastic muscles through their full ROM. (This is called passive stretching; the slow stretching does not elicit the spastic response.) However, passive stretching is no longer recommended in isolation. The current evidence places a greater emphasis on other methods of stretching, including positioning, orthoses, casting,* and especially active movement, where this is possible. The aim is to keep full ROM for as long as possible to prevent contractures from developing to the greatest possible extent. Working on ROM is not something that can begin when the child is older. It has to start right at the time of diagnosis. However, despite best efforts, it is often inevitable that some contractures may develop.

The rate of development of contractures often mirrors the rate of growth of the child; that is, contractures tend to develop during periods of rapid growth (which is why keeping a growth chart is useful). While great attention needs to be paid to stretching and activity during periods of active growth, stretching is needed throughout childhood and adolescence. Even in the "quieter" growth years, the child will still gain height.

Note that the situation is even more complicated, as it is actually possible that some muscles become too long in response to abnormal postures and movement.

b) Atypical bone development

Atypical bone development is interlinked with atypical muscle growth in spastic quadriplegia. The long bones of the body (the bones of the upper and lower limbs) grow in a particular area called the "growth plates" (see Figure 2.5.4), but it is the forces acting on the bones that play a part in their ultimate shape—termed "bone modeling."[132]

---

* Casting consists of stretching a muscle by applying a plaster of paris or a fiberglass cast; for example, a below-knee cast to stretch the tight gastrocnemius and/or soleus muscles (calf muscles) to hold the muscle in a position of maximum stretch. After a few days to one week, the cast can be removed. A series of casts is typically needed to gain the desired effect.

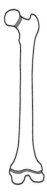

Figure 2.5.4 Growth plates (orange) in a long bone.

Growing bone is "plastic," or "malleable," which is what allows the forces to model the bone. The expressions "If you put a twist on a growing bone, it will take the twist" and "Just as the twig is bent the tree's inclined" illustrate this concept.

If the muscle forces and bone forces are typical and occur at the correct time in development, then the final shape of the bone will be typical as well (e.g., the femoral head and the hip socket helping to shape each other). If forces are atypical or mistimed in relation to a child's development, the bones may be misshaped.

The movements that help the child achieve the six main gross motor milestones* described in Chapter 1 and the time in development at which they occur are part of the typical forces acting on the bones. It is important to understand that the bones of younger children are more malleable than the bones of older children. Frequently in spastic quadriplegia, the child is late or unable to achieve gross motor milestones. For example, when a child is late in achieving a milestone, the bones are at a different stage of development and can be less malleable with less ability to remodel or reshape in addition to the influences of altered muscle forces and tone. We can compare it to providing opportunities for our children: we have to provide them at the right time. Peekaboo will delight your six-month-old infant, but your six-year-old child will likely roll their eyes if you try to play peekaboo with them. In the presence of spastic quadriplegia, typical bone modeling (shaping) may not occur as the bone grows.

---

* The milestones are significant, but so are the movements leading up to the milestones.

c) Common muscle and bone problems in spastic quadriplegia

The effectiveness of the muscle to produce movement depends not only on the muscle but also on the shape and length of the bones and the position of the joints. We have already reviewed the muscle problems that develop with growth in children with CP. If the position or shape of the bone and joint are not correct, muscle action and movement are interfered with.

The following are examples of common muscle and bone problems in spastic quadriplegia. They include:

- Upper limb contractures
- Scoliosis
- Hip displacement (subluxation and dislocation)
- Windswept hips
- Lower limb contractures
- Bone health problems

These problems may exist in isolation or in combination and each is explained below.

> Levi has dealt with all these problems.

i) Upper limb contractures

The most common upper extremity contractures are at the elbow (elbow flexion; that is, bent), pronated forearm (the hand is in the palm down position), and at the wrist (wrist flexion). (See Figure 2.5.5.) Contractures can also happen at the shoulders, and usually are such that the arm is locked close toward the middle of the body.

We saw earlier that the combination of the muscle, tendon, and other structures is collectively known as the muscle-tendon unit (MTU). The contracture occurs in the MTU and/or capsule of the joint, not just the muscle. Upper limb (and lower limb) contractures are complex to improve surgically. This is why a flexed wrist or elbow may not be resolved entirely with muscle or tendon lengthening surgery alone.

Sometimes, however, if the contractures are interfering with positioning or care, muscle or tendon lengthening surgery may be considered to achieve limited improved range of motion (ROM),* even if full ROM cannot be achieved.

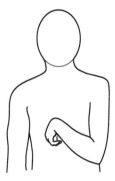

Figure 2.5.5 Flexed elbow, pronated forearm, and flexed wrist.

Levi has contractures in his thumbs. He has full range of motion in his arms, but they are typically held tight against his torso.

ii) Scoliosis
Scoliosis is a three-dimensional rotation and curvature of the spine. When viewed from the back, the spine of a person with scoliosis is a C-shaped curve instead of a straight line. See Figure 2.5.6.

---

* ROM, also called range of movement, is a measure of joint flexibility. The actual ROM through which a joint can be passively moved is measured in degrees. An instrument called a goniometer is used to measure the ROM of a joint.

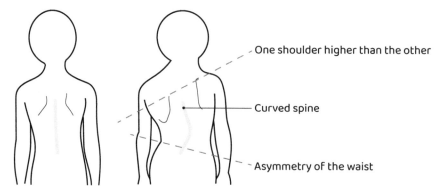

One shoulder higher than the other

Curved spine

Asymmetry of the waist

Figure 2.5.6 A typical spine (left) and a spine with scoliosis (right, showing a C-shaped curve). Note that one shoulder is higher than the other and there is asymmetry at the waist.

The angle of the scoliosis curve, the Cobb angle (also referred to as the curve magnitude) is measured on an X-ray image. The Cobb angle is the angle between the two most tilted vertebrae[*] at the upper and lower ends of a spinal curve (see Figure 2.5.7). A diagnosis of scoliosis is made when the Cobb angle is 10 degrees or greater. The Cobb angle is also used to monitor scoliosis progression and to guide treatment recommendations.

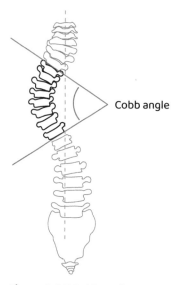

Cobb angle

Figure 2.5.7 Cobb angle measurement.

---

[*] The spine consists of vertebrae (the plural of vertebra) and intervertebral discs. Vertebrae are bony structures with a hole in the middle for the spinal cord to pass through.

The prevalence and severity of scoliosis in individuals with CP (all types) increases with GMFCS level.[133,134] The prevalence of scoliosis was found to be:[134]

- 71 percent for GMFCS level IV
- 79 percent for GMFCS level V

Untreated scoliosis can negatively impact an individual's quality of life and daily function, such as the ability to comfortably sit in a wheelchair or hold the body upright without assistance.[135] Scoliosis can cause one hip to be higher than the other (termed "pelvic obliquity") in sitting and standing. This results in more pressure being placed on the lower hip, buttock, and thigh while sitting. (See Figure 2.5.8.) Over time, this prolonged increase in pressure can cause physical discomfort, pain, pressure ulcers,* and intolerance to sitting. For individuals who were previously capable of some independent movement, scoliosis can decrease their ability to stand, walk, or participate in transfers. Large scoliosis curves also can negatively impact the lungs.

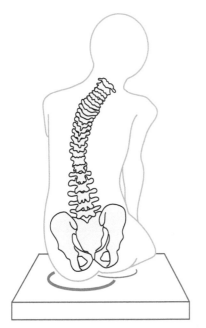

Figure 2.5.8 Pelvic obliquity in sitting.

---

* Areas of damaged skin and underlying tissue caused by prolonged pressure on the skin. Also known as bedsores, pressure wounds, or pressure sores.

Levi's scoliosis was first noted when he was about 11, in 2019. We were able to put off intervention until 2022. Levi's spinal fusion* was performed right before his lung function was affected. His lung health played a big role in deciding to intervene when we did.

iii) Hip displacement (subluxation and dislocation)

The hip joint is a ball-and-socket joint that is formed by the head (ball) of the femur and the acetabulum (socket) of the pelvis. Under the influence of bone growth and spastic muscles, a child's hip may become displaced: the ball moves partially out of the socket. This can be progressive and can lead to complete displacement. There are two stages of hip displacement:

- **Subluxated hip (hip subluxation)** is when the ball is partially out of the socket but is still in contact with it—the ball is still partially covered by the socket.
- **Dislocated hip (hip dislocation)** is when the ball has moved completely out of the socket.

The development of hip displacement is a slow process. Even though it starts out silently (it is painless), it can lead to pain and reduced function in the longer term. See Figure 2.5.9.

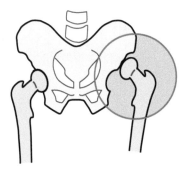

Figure 2.5.9 A dislocated hip. The right hip is normal. The left hip is dislocated: the head of the femur (ball) has moved completely out of the acetabulum (socket) of the pelvis.

---

* Spinal fusion involves fusing (joining together) two or more vertebrae in the spine to stop curve progression and reduce the size of the scoliosis curve.

Research has shown that the risk of hip displacement increases with GMFCS level.[136,137] The risk for children with CP has been found to be:

- 69 percent for GMFCS level IV
- 90 percent for GMFCS level V

The measure used in X-rays for hip surveillance (monitoring) is called the "migration percentage" (MP), also known as the Reimer's migration index (RMI). Both terms refer to the percentage of the ball that has moved out of the socket, which can range from 0 to 100. "Normal" is less than 10 percent,[3] and hip displacement (subluxation) is anything greater than that. Mild abnormalities may not be problematic, but once the MP is greater than 30 percent, the likelihood of further displacement is almost certain (if there is growth remaining). Hip dislocation is defined as MP over 90 and up to 100 percent.[138]

You may also come across the term "dysplasia," which means abnormal growth. Though closely related to hip displacement, it is not the same thing. Acetabular dysplasia is when the hip socket doesn't develop correctly and becomes shallow. It both results from and contributes to hip displacement.

iv) Windswept hips

Windswept hips comprise abduction and external rotation of one hip, with the opposite hip in adduction and internal rotation.* The posture derives its name from its appearance, as if the person's body had been blown that direction by a strong wind. Windswept hips interfere with supported standing potential and comfort in lying and sitting.[139]

---

* Hip abduction is movement of the thigh away from the midline. Hip external rotation is rotary movement of the thigh away from the midline. Hip adduction is movement of the thigh toward the midline. Hip internal rotation is rotary movement of the thigh toward the midline.

Levi has windswept hips. This has become more evident as he has grown, and we have made some adjustments to his wheelchair to prevent any sores due to his foot resting on the metal bar of his wheelchair footrest.

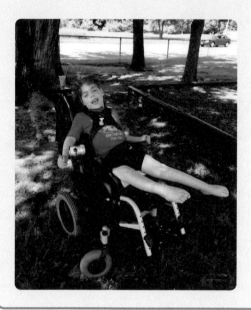

iv) Lower limb contractures

The most common lower limb contractures are flexed and adducted hips, flexed knees, and equinovarus or equinovalgus feet. See Table 2.5.1.

v) Bone health

Bone is a living tissue that is constantly being created, removed, and replaced. The term "osteoporosis" means "porous bones" (i.e., bones with low bone density). Low bone density arises when either insufficient new bone is created or the rate of absorption of bone is greater than the rate of formation.

As people age, more bone is naturally lost than replaced. People with osteoporosis, however, have greater bone loss than is normal for their age. Figure 2.5.10 shows a normal bone and one with osteoporosis; the latter has much less bone material (i.e., less bone density).

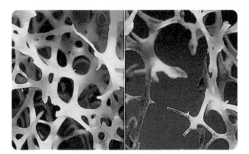

Figure 2.5.10 Cross-section of normal (left) and osteoporotic bone (right). Reproduced from Wikipedia user Gtirouflet, used under a Creative Commons license.

Bones can become so weak that a break (fracture) may occur with stress (such as a fall). A break may even occur spontaneously. Osteoporosis is a "silent" disease in that it is often diagnosed only when a bone fracture occurs. It is the most common cause of bone fractures among elderly people.

"Osteopenia" is the term used to define bone density that is not normal but not as low as in osteoporosis.[140] It can be regarded as the midpoint between healthy bone and osteoporosis. Having osteopenia places a person at risk of developing osteoporosis.

Low bone density is a serious problem in children with CP who are nonambulatory (not able to walk).[141]

Tertiary problems

The tertiary problems in spastic quadriplegia are the coping responses or compensations that arise in response to the individual's need to deal with or get around the primary and secondary problems.[132] For example, a compensation may develop where nonuse of the most affected arm is replaced by use of their mouth, legs, or any other body part or environmental support to complete a bilateral (two-handed) task or to avoid bilateral tasks altogether.

To correct the tertiary problems, the root cause (i.e., the primary and secondary problems), not the compensation, needs to be addressed.

Key points Chapter 2

- Spastic quadriplegia involves the upper and the lower limbs and trunk. The degree of involvement often varies between the upper and the lower limbs and between the two sides of the body.
- The majority of children with spastic quadriplegia are at levels IV and V for functional mobility (GMFCS) and for ability to handle objects (MACS).
- The most common causes of spastic quadriplegia are hypoxic ischemic encephalopathy, periventricular leukomalacia, and central nervous system infections.
- A useful framework for classifying the neuromusculoskeletal problems that occur in children with spastic CP categorizes them into primary, secondary, and tertiary problems.
- Primary problems are caused by the brain injury and are therefore present from when the brain injury occurred.
- Secondary problems develop over time in the growing child. They are problems of atypical muscle growth and bone development, and are referred to as "growth problems."
- Tertiary problems are the "coping responses" that arise to compensate for or counteract the primary and secondary problems.
- Spasticity is the most common type of atypical tone present in individuals with spastic quadriplegia, with 48 percent having co-occurring dyskinesia, and 3 percent having co-occurring hypotonia.
- A majority of children with spastic quadriplegia (all GMFCS levels) have associated problems varying from mild to severe in the areas of speech, intelligence (cognition), vision, and epilepsy. However, hearing is unaffected in many. Half have two or more severe associated problems.
- Prioritizing management of spastic quadriplegia begins with assuring general health, followed by addressing developmental progress and maximizing function, musculoskeletal health, and increasing participation.
- Common muscle and bone problems in spastic quadriplegia include upper limb contractures, scoliosis, hip displacement (subluxation/dislocation), windswept hips, lower limb contractures, and bone health problems.

Chapter 3

General health

Introduction

In the middle of difficulty lies opportunity.
Albert Einstein

This chapter addresses general health considerations across body systems. While each is addressed separately, they are intricately interlinked and interdependent. The body operates as a unified entity.

This chapter (and subsequent chapters) may feel daunting, particularly for a family with a child newly diagnosed with spastic quadriplegia. It is written to educate—never to alarm. Some sections may not apply to all readers.

USEFUL WEB RESOURCES

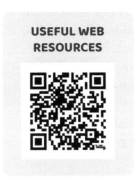

Respiratory system

Inhale the future, exhale the past.

Anonymous

It's no surprise that healthy lung function is vital to overall health. The lungs supply oxygen to the blood so that the cells of the body can get the oxygen they need. This is why the lung is called a "vital" organ. Supplying oxygen to the body requires healthy and strong lungs. The requirements for breathing and healthy and strong lungs include:

- Head and trunk positioning to allow for easy movement of air in and out.
- An open and clear airway (which includes the nose, mouth, throat, and lungs). Any blockages in the airway can cause breathing difficulties.
- Strong respiratory muscles for breathing, but also for coughing to clear the airway.
- Sufficient surface area and functional alveoli (tiny air sacs in the lungs) to allow the exchange of oxygen and carbon dioxide.

Respiratory conditions frequently arise in individuals with spastic quadriplegia for many reasons, including the following:

- They may have difficulty clearing their airway through coughing because of their abnormal tone and muscle weakness.
- They are at high risk of **sialorrhea** (excess saliva) and **drooling** (excess saliva dropping uncontrollably from the mouth), which may then be aspirated* which can lead to respiratory problems.
- They are at high risk of aspirating generally—food, liquids, and other secretions, in addition to saliva.
- They are at an increased risk for developing asthma. At least 1 in 5 children with CP have asthma compared with 1 in 12 typically developing peers.[142]

Because of the above difficulties with airway clearance paired with higher rates of aspiration and asthma, **obstructive lung conditions**, caused by blocked airflow, can arise putting individuals at risk of recurrent lung infections and chronic inflammation.

In addition, **restrictive lung conditions**, caused by a decrease in total air volume in the lungs, can arise due to contractures and progressive scoliosis.[143] Untreated, severe, scoliosis can impact respiratory function in two distinct ways:

- The curving and rotating of the spine can limit the amount of space the lungs have to expand and fill with air, making it difficult to breathe or cough to clear the airways, especially during illness.
- Postural problems can hamper the diaphragm's ability to move the abdominal contents downwards, thus limiting the ability of the lungs to expand.

Respiratory issues are the most common cause of morbidity (temporary or permanent disability) or mortality (death) in individuals with CP.[144] Novak and colleagues reported aspiration resulting in respiratory complication as a leading cause of death in individuals with CP.[14] Thus, diligent management of the respiratory system is of utmost importance in maintaining overall health.

The good news is that there are a variety of treatments that can help to improve respiratory function and decrease the risk of respiratory illness. Having a pulmonologist as part of the care team is invaluable as

---

* Food or liquid entering the airway instead of the esophagus.

they can develop a comprehensive treatment plan that includes preventing problems with lung function as well as an action plan for when the lung function is becoming challenged.

- **Sialorrhea treatment:** Sialorrhea becomes a concern when the saliva is aspirated and then contributes to problems with respiratory health. When sialorrhea is causing aspiration concerns, it may help to decrease the saliva volume, which can be achieved with medications administered orally (by mouth), enterally (directly to the gastrointestinal tract through a feeding tube), buccally (placed in the cheek area), or via a transdermal patch (skin patch). Botulinum neurotoxin A (BoNT-A) injection into the salivary glands has been shown to be effective at reducing saliva.[145] If the issue is drooling, that is more a cause of social concerns and skin irritation, and for those reasons, sialorrhea may also be treated, using the same medications.
- **Suctioning:** Suctioning is a method of removing secretions to clear the airway. It can be done with a flexible catheter passed through the nose or mouth. Suctioning can sometimes cause the individual to gag or vomit, so careful attention should be given to safe positioning and gentle yet effective suction pressure levels.
- **Cough assist device:** A cough assist device typically consists of a handheld device with a face mask or mouthpiece. The device applies positive pressure to the airway, then rapidly shifts to negative pressure.* This pressure change in the airway mimics a natural cough and helps to clear secretions for individuals who have a weak natural cough.
- **Inhaled or nebulized treatments:** An inhaler or nebulizer is commonly used to administer saline solution or mucolytic medications, which help break down mucus and ease airway clearance when combined with effective coughing, suctioning, or a cough assist device.
  - An inhaler is a small, handheld device that turns liquids into a fine spray (aerosol; i.e., droplets dispersed in air) that can then be inhaled through a mouthpiece while pushing a pump. It can be paired with a spacer (a chamber that can hold medication) for gradual inhalation (breathing in).

---

* Positive pressure creates a pushing effect in the airways that helps to expand the lungs and move mucus or secretions toward the mouth for coughing or spitting out. Negative pressure is like a suctioning effect that helps to pull mucus or secretions from the smaller airways into the larger ones, aiding in their removal.

○   A nebulizer is an electric machine that turns liquids into a fine spray that can then be inhaled through a mouthpiece or face mask. When hand-eye coordination is problematic, a nebulizer is preferable.

Other medications that may be administered using an inhaler or nebulizer include corticosteroids (anti-inflammatory medication) or bronchodilators (medication that relaxes the muscles around the airway to widen it). For children with CP who also have asthma, these are often given regularly as maintenance treatments and more frequently during times of illness.

- **Manual chest physiotherapy:** Manual chest physiotherapy is performed to loosen secretions from the chest wall through external manipulation of the thorax (chest) by applying percussion (tapping) and vibration (gentle shaking) techniques[146] in positions that promote drainage.

- **High-frequency chest wall compression therapy:** Also termed "vest therapy," this involves wearing a vest connected to an air pulse generator. The air pulses produced by the generator cause the vest to vibrate at high frequencies, loosening secretions from the chest wall. These loosened secretions can then be cleared through effective coughing, suctioning, or using a cough assist device.

- **Assisted ventilation:** This is the use of an external device to help with natural breathing. Assisted ventilation can be noninvasive or invasive and offers a high level of respiratory support.

  ○   **Noninvasive assistive ventilation:** Continuous positive airway pressure (CPAP) and bilevel positive airway pressure (BiPAP) machines are used for noninvasive assistive ventilation. A CPAP machine connects to a face (or nasal) mask and provides continuous airway pressure to keep the airways open. It is commonly used during sleep to treat sleep apnea.* See Figure 3.2.1.

---

* A sleep disorder characterized by pauses in breathing or shallow breaths during sleep, leading to disrupted sleep and possible health complications.

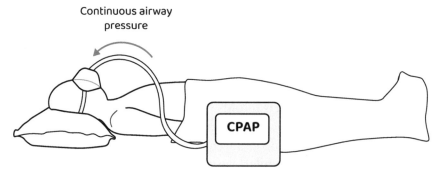

Figure 3.2.1 CPAP machine.

A BiPAP machine delivers high and low pressure to mimic breathing in and out. It makes breathing easier and can be used during the day or night. See Figure 3.2.2.

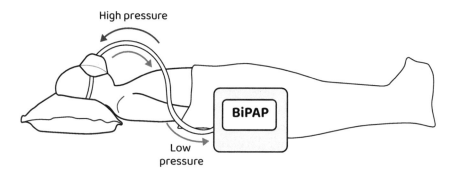

Figure 3.2.2 BiPAP machine.

○ **Invasive assisted ventilation:** A tracheostomy tube allows for invasive assisted ventilation. A tracheostomy is a surgical procedure in which a small opening is created in the windpipe (trachea), and a tube (tracheostomy tube) is placed in the opening. Ventilation devices can be connected to this tube to support breathing. See Figure 3.2.3.

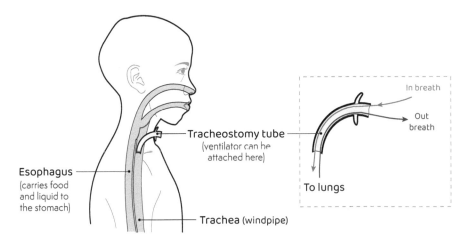

Figure 3.2.3 Tracheostomy tube.

The American Academy for Cerebral Palsy and Developmental Medicine (AACPDM) has published two care pathways: "Sialorrhea in Cerebral Palsy" and "Respiratory Health in Cerebral Palsy." Links to both are included in **Useful web resources.**

Levi's lung function was great until he began to hit puberty. His increasing scoliosis meant that his lung function might be impacted unless we intervened and agreed to spinal surgery. Around this time, his ability to come out of surgery with good lung function also decreased. He needed to be intubated* much longer than previously, and even needed CPAP and oxygen, which had never been an issue when he was younger. Lung function was a main decision point for doing spine surgery.

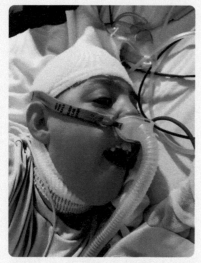

Levi with a nasal mask connecting to his CPAP machine.

---

* Intubation involves inserting a tube through the mouth or nose into the windpipe (trachea) to maintain an open airway, usually as a temporary measure.

Feeding, swallowing, and nutrition

Let food be thy medicine and medicine be thy food.
Hippocrates

Feeding refers to the process of consuming food or liquid. **Swallowing** refers to moving food or liquid down the throat, and **nutrition** refers to the process of getting nourishment necessary for health and growth. Growth is demanding work and requires energy, and optimal nutrition is key for growth.

Recall that the growth of children with spastic quadriplegia is less than typical peers. Individuals with spastic quadriplegia often have challenges with feeding and swallowing, which can give rise to nutritional challenges. Optimal nutrition is also key for health. For example, malnutrition is a key risk factor for the development of pressure ulcers and poor wound healing.[147] Recurrent illnesses can affect nutrition and growth. Thus, optimal nutrition, health, and growth are closely interlinked. Thankfully, many resources exist to ensure optimal nutrition to maximize growth and health.

Malnutrition and undernutrition are not exactly the same. "Malnutrition" is the broader term that includes both undernutrition (inadequate intake of nutrients, including essential nutrients) and overnutrition (excessive intake of nutrients). Children and adolescents with spastic quadriplegia are at risk of both. Changes in a child's skin, hair, or nails can indicate a deficiency of essential nutrients.[148]

Mealtimes can sometimes be very lengthy and tiring for the person with spastic quadriplegia—it takes energy to eat food—and they can be a struggle for the caregiver. The Eating and Drinking Classification System (EDACS) addressed in section 1.7 classifies individuals based on their eating and drinking ability from the perspectives of safety (aspiration—food or liquid entering the airway or lungs instead of the esophagus, and choking—blockage of the airway by food) and efficiency (amount of food and liquid lost from the mouth and time taken to eat) and is helpful when planning appropriate management strategies.

This section addresses:

- Feeding and swallowing challenges
- A philosophical note on feeding
- Measuring height and weight
- Weight management
- Interventions for feeding, swallowing, and nutrition challenges
- Oral hygiene and dental care

Feeding and swallowing challenges

A basic understanding of feeding and swallowing is useful here. Feeding and swallowing can be divided into three phases (see Figure 3.3.1):[149]

- **Oral phase:** The oral phase (phase relating to the mouth) involves sucking, chewing, and moving food into the throat (pharynx).
- **Pharyngeal phase:** The pharyngeal phase (phase relating to the throat) involves starting the swallow and moving food down the throat and protecting the airway to keep food and liquid out.
- **Esophageal phase:** During the esophageal phase (phase relating to the esophagus—the tube connecting the pharynx and stomach), the

food moves into the esophagus, which squeezes food down into the stomach and prevents stomach contents from coming back up.

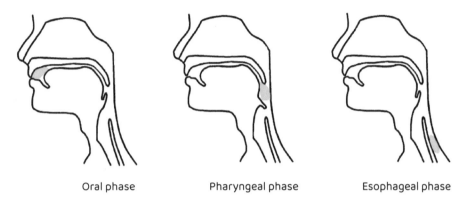

Oral phase	Pharyngeal phase	Esophageal phase

Figure 3.3.1 The three phases of feeding and swallowing. Reproduced from Analysis of swallowing in infants and adults using speckle pattern analysis, by R. Shahmoom et al. (2022). *Springer Nature.* Used under a Creative Commons Attribution 4.0 International License. https://creativecommons.org/licenses/by/4.0/

Individuals with spastic quadriplegia may struggle with any of these three phases as they all depend on motor coordination of the muscles of chewing and swallowing, and sensation of the food or liquid in the mouth, pharynx, and esophagus:

- Problems with the oral phase may include challenges with sucking, eating from a spoon, chewing, or drinking from a cup.[149] For instance, some foods require more strength to chew and the movements to move food from the teeth to the back and sides of the mouth may be difficult.
- Problems with the pharyngeal phase include difficulties with swallowing, such as mistimed swallowing that can lead to aspirating food or liquid, or to choking. Recall that individuals with spastic quadriplegia may also experience sialorrhea (excess saliva). When sialorrhea is paired with dysphagia (swallowing disorders), an individual may aspirate their saliva, or they may choke. Recognition and management of dysphagia is extremely important since aspiration resulting in respiratory complications is a leading cause of mortality in individuals with CP.[14]
- Problems with the esophageal phase may involve the transit of food or liquids, which may be slower or may lead to reflux (food or liquids

moving in the wrong direction, from stomach to esophagus or from esophagus into the airway).[148] When stomach contents move back into the esophagus, this is referred to as gastroesophageal reflux (GER).

Signs of a feeding or swallowing disorder may be obvious, such as choking, coughing, or gagging while eating. However, the signs may be less obvious such as a hoarse or breathy voice after mealtime, refusal to eat, or recurrent respiratory infections.[149]

Section 4.2, under Speech and Language Pathology, addresses dysphagia (swallowing disorders) therapy; in particular, diagnosis and treatment for aspiration concerns.

A philosophical note on feeding

Immediately following the infant's first breath, the mission of the parents is to feed the child. It is an innate drive of parents to assure nutrition for their children. For this reason, the work of feeding is emotionally connected to the perceived success of parenting: "I feed my child, therefore, I am a successful parent." As a result, when a child is struggling to eat as a result of their CP, their parents may incorrectly feel a sense of failure: "I cannot feed my child, therefore I have failed to meet their needs as a parent."

It is important to understand that the process of feeding, swallowing, and getting good nutrition is a surprisingly complex task that most of us take for granted. When the nervous system and the many coordinated muscles for feeding, swallowing, and processing food for nutrition are challenged and do not operate well and efficiently, feeding can quickly become a struggle for the person with spastic quadriplegia and their dedicated parents. It is imperative that parents understand that there are very often neuromuscular problems challenging feeding for a child with spastic quadriplegia. There can also be sensory issues in relation to the types of food that the child can manage and the viscosity of liquids they can drink.

Challenges with feeding, swallowing, and nutrition may be present in infants, or they may not arise until the child begins eating solid food and struggles with the more complex movements required for chewing and swallowing, along with the endurance needed for the increased calorie intake as they grow in size. As well, problems can evolve over time. A child who was once able to eat and drink without issue may begin to have problems as they grow and are impacted by some of the secondary problems, discussed above, that come with spastic quadriplegia. Ongoing assessment and evaluation of feeding, swallowing and nutrition are important.

Measuring height and weight

Obtaining accurate height and weight for individuals with spastic quadriplegia can be difficult for a number of reasons, including inability to stand, presence of scoliosis, and presence of contractures. Height may be obtained by measuring segments of the body and adding them together to get an overall height, or by measuring the length of segments of the body (e.g., tibia, knee, or forearm) and then estimating overall height from these values. Weight can be obtained using a wheelchair scale, a specialized device that accommodates both the wheelchair and the child. The process involves placing the wheelchair with the child onto the scale, then removing the child from the wheelchair, and weighing the empty wheelchair. The weight of the wheelchair is subtracted from the total to derive the child's weight. A similar method that can be used for a small child is to weigh the child with the parent holding them, followed by the parent alone, and subtracting to get the weight of the child.

Weight management

While many children and adolescents with spastic quadriplegia struggle to maintain an appropriate weight and are often underweight, others can be overweight or obese. There are many factors that contribute to challenges in maintaining appropriate body mass index (BMI).* Individuals may be underweight because of inadequate caloric intake due to feeding issues as described above or because of excessive energy

---

* BMI is calculated by dividing a person's body mass in kilograms by the square of their body height in meters.

use as their movement may not be as energy efficient as their typically developing peers (due to musculoskeletal problems) thus placing an extra demand on calorie intake. Individuals who use feeding tubes (addressed further in this section) can become overweight or obese if the calorie intake is higher than required. Either overweight or obesity may develop in those even without feeding tubes due to lack of movement. A study of nutritional status found that most cases of moderate to severe undernutrition occurred in those at GMFCS level V, while most cases of overweight and obesity occurred in those at GMFCS level IV.[150]

Weight management is also important to protect the well-being and health of caregivers since almost all individuals with GMFCS level IV or V require significant assistance with movement and transfers.

Interventions for feeding, swallowing, and nutrition challenges

The following is an explanation of different interventions for feeding, swallowing, and nutrition challenges. They include:

a) **Oral feeding**
b) **Enteral feeding**
   - **Nasogastric tube (NG tube)**
   - **Gastrostomy tube (G-tube)**
   - **Jejunostomy tube (J-tube)**
   - **Gastrojejunostomy tube (G-J-tube)**

a) Oral feeding

Oral feeding is food and drink taken by mouth. If oral feeding is impaired due to swallowing challenges, or if it is so inefficient that it takes too long to consume adequate calories, a consultation with speech and occupational therapists (ideally in a multidisciplinary feeding clinic) may be helpful. Oral motor therapy may assist with developing skills required for feeding. If this does not advance nutritional intake, further intervention may be needed.

Further intervention could include changing the consistency of foods. For example, food can be pureed to make it easier, safer, and less energy consuming to swallow. Or liquids can be thickened to allow for safe swallowing and to avoid aspiration when slower transit of the liquid is needed. Supplementing feeding with high-calorie shakes and other foods by mouth may be introduced. In addition, adaptive devices such as specialized utensils and cups can be helpful.

b) Enteral feeding

Enteral feeding (also known as tube-feeding) is liquid nutrition delivered via a feeding tube, a plastic tube that delivers nutrition directly into the stomach or small intestine. When feeding and swallowing challenges interfere with safe or efficient mealtimes, the multidisciplinary team may recommend a feeding tube to supplement the nutrition that can be taken in orally.

Parents are cautioned to avoid perceiving the recommendation of a feeding tube as their failure to meet the child's needs. Rather, the choice to supplement intake with enteral feeding can be a real gift. For the child who is struggling to feed and is uncomfortable or fatigued with feeding, or the child whose days are spent constantly trying to eat enough calories, feeding tube supplementation may relieve discomfort, preserve energy, and allow time for more fully participating in life.

The individual can still eat and drink conventionally as long as it is safe; the feeding tube supplements their diet to ensure adequate calorie intake. Supplemental tube-feeding may support as little as 10 percent or as much as 100 percent of calorie intake. Physicians and dietitians work together with the individual and their family to determine how much and when tube-feeding should be provided for supplementation. Although it is uncommon to do so, a feeding tube can be removed if is no longer necessary.

Feeding tube options include:

- **Nasogastric tube (NG tube):** A tube inserted through the nose that carries nutrition to the stomach. Nutrition is delivered by syringe (see Figure 3.3.2) or by pump.

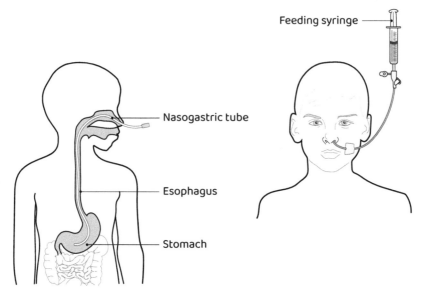

Figure 3.3.2 Nasogastric tube (NG tube)

- **Gastrostomy tube (G-tube):** A tube surgically inserted to carry nutrition to the stomach. Inside the stomach a balloon is inflated to prevent the tube from falling out. A full meal can be delivered at once by G-tube, usually via gravity feed from a bag, and the stomach will then slowly move the meal into the small intestine. See Figure 3.3.3. (Note that the terms "G-tube" and "PEG"* can be used interchangeably.)

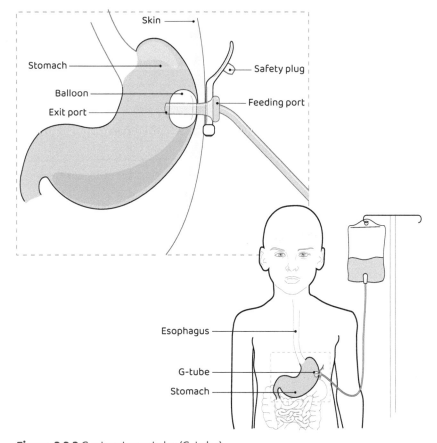

Figure 3.3.3 Gastrostomy tube (G-tube)

---

* "PEG" is percutaneous endoscopic gastrostomy. "Percutaneous" means through the skin; "endoscopic" refers to a technique in which a flexible camera is placed through the mouth into the stomach to visualize the best place for the tube; "gastrostomy" is a procedure for creating an opening into the stomach from the abdominal wall.[151]

- **Jejunostomy tube (J-tube):** A tube surgically inserted to carry nutrition to the jejunum (a section of the small intestine). Inside the jejunum, a balloon is inflated to prevent the tube from falling out. A meal must be delivered slowly through the J-tube (usually dripped via a pump) as the small intestine cannot tolerate a whole meal at once. See Figure 3.3.4.

  A J-tube may be preferable if, for example, feeding difficulties include gastroesophageal reflux disease (GERD)* or vomiting such that G-tube feedings are poorly tolerated.

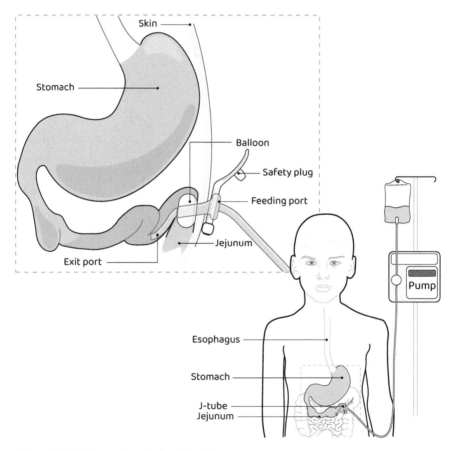

Figure 3.3.4 Jejunostomy tube (J-tube)

---

* Gastroesophageal reflux (GER) occurs when stomach contents flow in the wrong direction; that is, from the stomach back into the esophagus. GER is also referred to as "acid indigestion," "acid reflux," "acid regurgitation," "heartburn," and simply "reflux." Gastroesophageal reflux disease (GERD) occurs when GER is more severe and long-lasting.

- **Gastrojejunostomy tube (G-J-tube):** Two tubes in one, surgically inserted with one tube routing to the stomach (G) and the other to the jejunum (J). Inside the stomach, a balloon is inflated to prevent the tube from falling out. A G-J-tube is used when there is potential benefit from both stomach and small intestine access for delivering nutrition. See Figure 3.3.5.

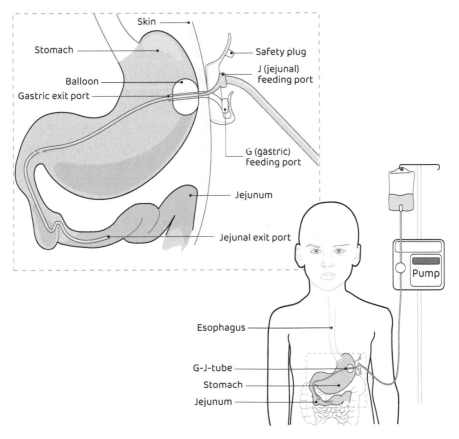

Figure 3.3.5 Gastrojejunostomy tube (G-J-tube). Here, a meal is being delivered through the J port of the G-J-tube.

Among these feeding tube types, an NG tube is considered a short-term nutrition option, while a G-tube, J-tube, or G-J-tube is typically recommended if supplemental nutrition is expected to be needed for longer than six weeks.[152]

A G-tube is the most common feeding tube option. It is generally preferred over a J-tube because it allows food to enter the body at an earlier stage in digestion and can take a large quantity of food at once, as opposed to being delivered as a slow drip feed. A G-tube thus allows feeding time to be shorter.

There is evidence supporting the use of feeding tubes. Recall section 2.5, which showed that both boys and girls with CP GMFCS level V who were tube-fed had better growth than those fed orally.[109,110]

Levi has a feeding tube for all his nutrition. He had it placed after he was ill with his *Salmonella* Paratyphii infection and stopped drinking. We did try feeding therapy for a summer, but Levi's inability to coordinate his swallow made it frustrating and time consuming. His short bowel status also complicates his nutritional status. The feeding tube is a blessing, especially as Levi needs so many daily medications and they can all be put through the tube. He does not have to swallow any of them. We can also increase water intake when he is dehydrated.

We still sometimes do tastes of foods, but Levi doesn't seem to have any interest in food.

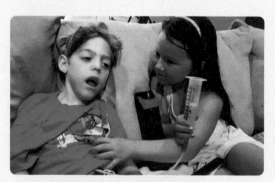
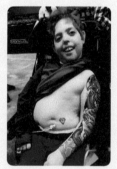
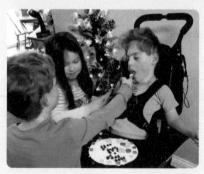

Cam (left), Ana (middle), and Levi (right).

Oral hygiene and dental care

Related to the issues of feeding and swallowing is the need for oral hygiene and regular dental care. They are of great importance for those with spastic quadriplegia, but they can be challenging. Brushing teeth and flossing twice daily can be difficult to accomplish completely and thoroughly. Jaw-clenching muscle spasms and trouble with motor control to open the mouth and maintain it open for brushing can interfere with complete oral care. A sensitive gag reflex may interfere as well. Furthermore, some medications may contribute to dry mouth and put the person at even greater risk for tooth decay or oral infections, both of which can cause pain. Teeth grinding is also common, although often of no significant concern, in individuals with spastic quadriplegia.

These and other factors highlight the need for regular dental checkups. For an individual with limited ability to communicate, regular dental evaluations can address any sources of potential pain or other issues. To do a complete oral examination and cleaning, it is not uncommon for the dental team to put the individual under sedation so that the muscles of the jaw are relaxed and the whole oral cavity is available. Finding a dentist who works with this unique set of circumstances can be challenging, but establishing that relationship and maintaining it is important.

Digestive system

One cannot think well, love well, sleep well, if one has not dined well.

Virginia Woolf

In previous sections, we described challenges that individuals with spastic quadriplegia face with feeding and swallowing and how some can impact respiratory health. This section addresses the health and function of the digestive system, also known as the gastrointestinal (GI) system. The term "gastrointestinal" is derived from "gastro," meaning stomach, and "intestinal," meaning the intestines. Individuals with spastic quadriplegia often face digestive challenges that can cause pain, impact respiratory health, and contribute to other medical problems. Staying on top of digestive health is important for the overall health and quality of life of the individual with spastic quadriplegia.

The role of the digestive system is to take in and process food and liquids. A healthy digestive system needs to not only break the food down so that it can be converted to energy, but also to absorb nutrients as it moves the food along, disposing of any byproducts in the form of stool. Absorbing water is vitally important as well, as the body cannot survive without adequate fluid. The digestive system does its job of digesting food "automatically" under the control of the autonomic nervous system. The following subsections address common digestive system challenges among individuals with spastic quadriplegia, including:

- Gastroesophageal reflux
- Gastroesophageal reflux disease
- Slow gastric motility
- Slow intestinal motility
- Constipation
- Abdominal pain
- Bowel incontinence

Levi's digestive system is compromised not only by his CP but also because he lost 70 percent of his small intestine during the surgery to treat the necrotizing enterocolitis he acquired in the NICU. Levi's digestive system is the first place we get clues from that he is sick or has a cold. His stools are impacted immediately by any illness. Levi's gastroenterologist is amazing and an integral part of his complex care team!

Gastroesophageal reflux

Gastroesophageal reflux (GER) occurs when stomach contents flow in the wrong direction; that is, from the stomach back into the esophagus. Many people can have GER once in a while. GER is also referred to as acid indigestion, acid reflex, acid regurgitation, heartburn, and simply reflux.[153]

Gastroesophageal reflux disease

When GER is more severe and long-lasting, gastroesophageal reflux disease (GERD) can occur, which can lead to complications over time.[153] GERD can be caused by many factors, such as atypical activity of the muscles required to squeeze food from the pharynx into the esophagus (esophagus motility), atypical activity of the lower esophageal sphincter (the muscle that prevents stomach contents from moving back up into the esophagus), and atypical activity of the muscles required to empty the stomach contents into the intestines (gastric emptying).[154] The risk of developing GERD may be increased by prolonged lying down, and in individuals with CP, it can be a source of pain and can compromise respiratory health. It is commonly associated with scoliosis, seizures, and chronic respiratory disease.[154]

Common symptoms of GERD may include irritability, arching of the back, vomiting, refusal to eat, and coughing after meals. GERD can cause long-term complications such as esophagitis (inflammation of the esophagus), malnutrition, and recurrent respiratory infections.[154]

Evaluation for the presence of GERD is imperative if it is suspected. This usually begins with a careful review of symptoms and their timing in relation to feeding and positioning during feeding. This history provides clues to the care team about the likelihood of GERD being implicated in the symptoms. Based on history alone, if GERD is suspected, treatment with medication may be initiated. Medication is intended to either reduce acid production by the stomach or neutralize stomach acid. Tests that may be recommended include a pH test (a thin tube is inserted into the esophagus to measure acid level) or an upper endoscopy test. An upper endoscopy test is performed under anesthesia, and it involves a camera, also termed "scope," inserted into the esophagus for direct visualization of the esophagus, stomach, and the beginning of the small intestine. In some cases, a surgical procedure to tighten the lower esophageal sphincter may be recommended to limit the painful reflux. This is commonly referred to as a Nissen procedure or a Nissen fundoplication.

Levi had trouble with reflux as an infant. He vomited after nearly every feeding and consequently didn't gain weight.

During the surgery to place Levi's feeding tube, the doctors also did a procedure called a Nissen fundoplication, essentially tying Levi's stomach around his esophagus so he couldn't vomit. He doesn't vomit any longer, though he still retches once in a while. His feeding tube has been a lifesaver, not only on a daily basis but also when he is sick. If he is retching, we can empty his stomach contents through the tube, which allows him to be much more comfortable.

Slow gastric motility

"Gastric motility" refers to the contraction and relaxation of the muscles in the stomach walls, which help break down food into smaller particles and mix it with gastric juices for digestion. Slow gastric motility refers to the slow transit of food from the stomach into the small intestine and then the large intestine. Slow gastric motility can be challenging because it can contribute to nausea, vomiting, stomach pain, feeding intolerance, and/or constipation. Gastric motility problems can mimic some of the same symptoms of GERD, making it difficult to distinguish between the two.

For evaluation of gastric motility problems, again, the clinician begins with a detailed history. Evaluation may include a gastric motility or emptying study where food (or formula) is combined with a marker (a dye) that can be visualized on an X-ray. After food is taken by the individual (either orally or enterally), a series of X-rays are taken over time to follow how long it takes the stomach to pass the food into the small intestine. Probiotics* and medications may be helpful to improve gastric motility, and often adjusting the feeding regimen can help.

Slow intestinal motility

"Intestinal motility" refers to the contraction and relaxation of the muscles in the intestines (small and large), which move the food forward allowing further digestion, absorption of nutrients and water, and eventual elimination of waste. Slow intestinal motility can contribute to an easily upset stomach, GER, GERD, and constipation. Though dietary supplements or medications may be considered to improve intestinal motility, the evidence is weak regarding their ability to improve the symptoms of GER or GERD.[155]

---

* Live microorganisms introduced into the body for their beneficial effects.

Constipation

"Constipation" is defined as having fewer than three bowel movements in a week.[156] Other typical signs of constipation may include hard stools, difficulties or pain with stooling, and abdominal pain.

When constipation persists for several weeks or longer, it is known as chronic constipation, which often affects individuals with spastic quadriplegia.[157] In one study, constipation was reported in 72 percent of children with CP GMFCS levels IV and V.[158] Chronic constipation also contributes to increased GERD symptoms, nausea and vomiting, feeding intolerance, pain, and irritability. Chronic constipation makes it challenging to take in adequate nutrition and markedly impacts quality of life. In severe cases, chronic constipation can lead to fecal impaction and may require hospital admission to successfully clean out the bowels.

Constipation can be made worse by medications commonly prescribed (e.g., to treat seizures, pain, bladder dysfunction) and have been shown to slow the movement of food through the digestive system.[159] Some medications used to treat dystonia and sialorrhea can also contribute to constipation.

The optimal goal is to avoid constipation in individuals with spastic quadriplegia, with at least three bowel movements weekly that are soft, comfortable, and produce near full evacuation of the large intestine. To achieve this, it may help to incorporate into the diet fruits rich in sorbitol (a natural sugar) like prunes and pears, alongside fiber-rich foods and sufficient fluid. However, many individuals with spastic quadriplegia benefit from a prescribed bowel program that often includes stool softeners, laxatives, stool bulking agents, and commonly, a combination of these. When these supplements, taken orally or enterally, are still not sufficient to effect a regular bowel movement, suppositories to stimulate the evacuation of stool, or enemas* to assist that evacuation, may be needed.

---

* **Suppositories** are small, solid, medicated preparations that are inserted into the rectum (final section of large intestine ending at the anus) to stimulate bowel movements. **Enemas** involve introducing a liquid into the rectum to soften the stool and facilitate bowel movements.

Another important constipation prevention technique is encouraging the individual to increase the time spent in an upright position; for example, by using a standing device.[157]

Abdominal pain

"Abdominal pain" refers to discomfort or distress experienced in the area between the chest and the pelvis, which includes various organs such as the stomach, liver, gallbladder, and intestines. "Stomach pain" specifically indicates discomfort in the stomach. Abdominal pain is a frequently reported concern in individuals with CP (all types).[160,161] It may be related to constipation, slow gastric or intestinal motility, or GERD, but it also may be of unclear cause.[161]

The source of abdominal pain or discomfort is frequently challenging to identify, partly because the discomfort can be nonspecific, vague, and intermittent. Questions to ask that help identify the source include:

- Is it relieved or exacerbated by feeding?
- Does changing the food or formula help?
- Is the pain relieved by passing gas or after having a bowel movement?
- Is the discomfort accompanied by increased spitting up or vomiting?

If there clearly is pain, but the individual is not able to communicate where the pain is located, a thorough review of the digestive system should be done to look for hidden causes, such as gallstones.*

Bowel incontinence

"Bowel incontinence" is a lack of voluntary control over bowel movements, and it is common in individuals with spastic quadriplegia. A UK study found that children with bilateral CP GMFCS levels IV and V achieved day and nighttime bowel and bladder (addressed in next section) continence more slowly and less completely than typically

---

* Tiny, hard masses that form in the gallbladder or bile ducts due to bile pigments, cholesterol, and calcium salts. They can cause severe pain and block bile ducts.

developing peers.[162] Attainment of continence was greater for those at GMFCS level IV than level V. See Table 3.4.1.

Bowel incontinence can be embarrassing, uncomfortable, and present many social challenges. However, the individual's care team can help limit the impact that this problem has on quality of life.

Table 3.4.1 Percentage of children with bilateral CP GMFCS levels IV and V achieving day and nighttime bowel and bladder continence

GMFCS LEVEL	PERCENTAGE ACHIEVING BOWEL CONTINENCE		PERCENTAGE ACHIEVING BLADDER CONTINENCE	
	By day	By night	By day	By night
IV	62% by age 5 years	50% by age 5 years	58% by age 5 years	50% by age 5 years
V	16% by age 6 years	12% by age 11 years	11% by age 6 years	12% by age 11 years

Individuals who are showing some progress in continence, but struggling to achieve success, may benefit from a consultation with a physical therapist who specializes in pelvic floor physical therapy. In addition, occupational therapists may recommend adaptive toileting equipment to help with positioning comfortably and safely on the commode. Another strategy that may be used to achieve bowel continence is timed toileting, in which the individual sits on the toilet about 30 minutes after a daily meal (e.g., 30 minutes after dinner) for up to 20 minutes, or until they achieve a bowel movement. If the individual is not able to control their bowels, this technique can be used in combination with a bowel program that includes a suppository or enema. This may allow a more predictable evacuation of the stool (that is, at the same time and in the same place daily).

In some cases, a procedure known as an antegrade continence enema (ACE) may be performed for more thorough and predictable evacuation of the stool. This is a surgical procedure to create a passageway between the large intestine and an opening in the lower abdomen. A catheter (tubing) is placed into the opening, and irrigation is given through the opening to flush out the stool through the rectum and into the toilet. This helps in the management of bowel incontinence and prevents constipation.

Levi is unable to assist with toileting, though we did attempt to potty train him when he was about three. He needed full support to sit on the toilet, and when he was too big to support, we stopped trying. He did not enjoy sitting on the toilet, as it was uncomfortable for him and painful to have a bowel movement. There were many tears involved, and he came to associate those bad feelings with the toilet.

Levi has always had issues with watery stools due to his short bowel. Interestingly, he has difficulty releasing his bowels to have a bowel movement. Even though he is not truly constipated, he still has discomfort during elimination.

Urinary system

Courage doesn't always roar. Sometimes courage is the little voice at
the end of the day that says I'll try again tomorrow.

Mary Anne Radmacher

Individuals with spastic quadriplegia may face challenges with urinary
incontinence (defined as a lack of voluntary control over urination),
and have increased difficulty with toilet training. Recall from the previous section that children with bilateral CP GMFCS levels IV and V
achieved day and nighttime bladder continence more slowly and less
completely than typically developing peers.[162] When we understand the
complex bodily processes of storing urine, sending a signal that the
bladder is full, holding onto urine, and finally releasing urine, we begin
to understand why this is hard for individuals with spastic quadriplegia.

Urinary continence begins with maturation of the communication
between the bladder and the brain—communication that happens first
along the sensory pathways from the bladder to areas of the brain that
perceive the bladder as "full." When the brain receives the message
that the bladder is full, the individual is able to maintain motor control
over the urinary sphincter in order to get to the toilet and release the

urine in a controlled fashion. In contrast, in infantile or immature and challenged bladder-to-brain communication, the bladder fills until the default sensors are tripped, and then empties spontaneously into the diaper. The bladder is not waiting for the brain to tell the sphincter to relax as it would in a mature bladder-to-brain communication.

Any challenges to the sensory and motor pathways between the bladder and brain can challenge toileting success. Furthermore, just as spasticity can affect the skeletal muscles, it can also affect the bladder muscles and those of the urinary system such that this high tone may interfere with urine storage, bladder sensation, and motor control for continence.

While incontinence is the most common urinary system problem, others may be present, such as the need to urinate frequently and urgently, hesitancy, and urinary retention.[163] Spasticity in the muscles of the urinary system and a small bladder capacity are some of the causes of urinary problems.[163]

Progress in toileting continence is delayed in individuals with spastic quadriplegia, and often strategies to help achieve and maintain that continence are needed. Timed toileting is an initial strategy that can be tried. It consists of helping the individual to the commode on a predictable schedule (for instance every two hours from waking until bedtime) to help them associate the sensation of a full bladder with the sensation of release of urine. This, potentially, allows them to achieve better motor control and therefore better continence. Physical therapists who specialize in pelvic floor physical therapy may be helpful, and occupational therapists may recommend adaptive toileting equipment to help with positioning comfortably and safely on the commode. This work is time and effort intensive for the individual with spastic quadriplegia and their caregivers, and for best success, the program should be standardized across all the individual's environments, such as home and school.

When the best efforts at toilet training are employed, but success is still elusive, a consultation with a pediatric urologist may be useful. Often this consultation will consist of obtaining an X-ray to evaluate the intestinal tract for constipation, which very often contributes to urinary incontinence. Other findings such as bladder or kidney stones may be identified, though less commonly. A renal ultrasound is usually taken to make sure the kidneys are not being impacted negatively by a chronically full bladder (urinary retention). A voiding cystourethrogram test may be recommended. This involves placing a urinary catheter into the bladder through the urethra to fill the bladder to its capacity. The amount of urine and pressure that the bladder can take gives information about its capacity to hold urine and its ability to release urine. Based on the results of the test, medications may be prescribed to more easily allow the bladder to hold onto urine or allow the sphincter to release urine.

Despite these challenges, a study found that 91 percent of individuals with spastic diplegia and quadriplegia (all GMFCS levels) with continence problems achieved continence with conservative care, which included a functional toileting review and medication.[164] Achieving urinary continence was found to be related to ability to communicate and environmental opportunity to succeed.

Epilepsy

The brain is the last and grandest biological frontier,
the most complex thing we have yet discovered in our universe.

James D. Watson

Epilepsy is a neurological disorder typically accompanied by seizures. A seizure is "uncontrolled, abnormal electrical activity of the brain that may cause changes in the level of consciousness, behavior, memory, or feelings."[165] Epilepsy is typically diagnosed after at least two unprovoked seizures, not stemming from any identifiable cause like fever, occurring more than 24 hours apart.[166]

Since epilepsy is due to abnormal brain activity and CP is caused by an injury to the brain, it would follow that epilepsy is more prevalent in individuals with CP than in the typical population. As we saw in section 2.1, an Australian study found that 53 percent of children age five with spastic quadriplegia (all GMFCS levels) have epilepsy.[80] The prevalence and severity of associated problems, including epilepsy, was found to be greater in children at higher GMFCS levels compared with those at lower GMFCS levels.[80] In addition, a European study found a higher prevalence of epilepsy among children with CP who have severe intellectual impairment, severe visual impairment, severe hearing impairment, or who are unable to walk.[167]

Seventy percent of children with CP and epilepsy experience the onset of seizures within the first year of life, which is younger than in a comparison group—children without CP but with epilepsy.[168] Children with CP who experience seizures in the neonatal period (defined as the first four weeks of life) are more likely to be diagnosed with epilepsy.[169] Although some types of seizures may be more common in individuals with CP, all seizure types may occur.[168] Since spastic quadriplegia is associated with injuries impacting larger areas of the brain, generalized seizures* often ensue.[170]

Information on the management of epilepsy in individuals with spastic quadriplegia is included in Appendix 3 (online).

When Levi was given his official diagnosis of spastic quadriplegia cerebral palsy (QSCP), I of course read up on the condition. As you know, that is not a delightful read. I was worried that my child would wind up with the variety of conditions that can often go along with QSCP, like epilepsy, feeding issues, speech problems, spine issues, etc. And that's what happened. Levi had his first tonic-clonic seizure at school when he was eight years old. Looking back, I believe it was induced by being overheated. At that point, no one knew Levi had epilepsy, so when he went into seizure, the teacher called 911 and he was taken to the hospital. (An added complication that day was that his wheelchair was left at school, making it difficult to get him home from the hospital.)

He was diagnosed with epilepsy and started medications to control the seizures. Levi's EEG† showed a constant low level of misfirings, though to date we have never seen an official seizure on any of his EEGs. Most of his epilepsy shows as erratic brain activity on the EEG monitor. He

---

* Seizures that result from abnormal activity within both halves of the brain. These often result in a loss of consciousness and may present as urgent situations, requiring immediate treatment.[171]

† EEG (electroencephalography) is a noninvasive test that records electrical activity in the brain using electrodes placed on the scalp.

does have a rescue med* in case he has a seizure that he doesn't come out of after five minutes. We have so far never needed it, though we have it attached to his wheelchair to be available.

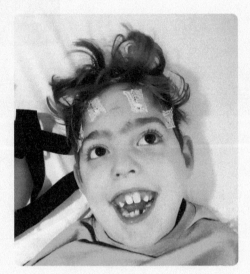

Levi having an EEG.

---

* A rescue med (medication), in the context of epilepsy, is a fast-acting medication given during a seizure to stop or shorten its length.

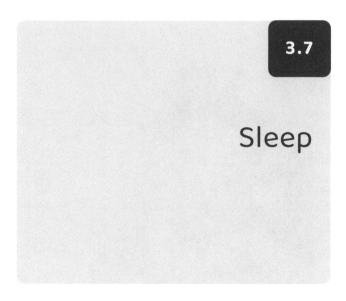

3.7

Sleep

We are such stuff as dreams are made on;
and our little life is rounded with a sleep.
William Shakespeare

Adequate sleep is necessary for brain development, and the disruption of sleep and sleep deprivation has been shown to impact emotional and cognitive functioning, impair overall quality of life, and lead to mental and behavioral health issues.[172,173] Untreated sleep problems can lead to poor alertness, daytime sleepiness, irritability, and poor participation, which can contribute to additional delays in development. They can further contribute to respiratory problems, already a concern in individuals with spastic quadriplegia.

Almost everyone experiences sleep deprivation at some point in their lives, and they are aware of the impact that this has on performance during the daytime.

Sleep disorders are common in individuals with CP. Seventy-two percent of children with CP GMFCS levels IV and V were reported to have sleep disorders.[158] More than half of children with spastic quadriplegia have epilepsy,[80] and children with CP and epilepsy are even more at risk for sleep disorders.[174]

Individuals with spastic quadriplegia may have problems both with falling asleep and staying asleep. Sleep problems can include sleep-related breathing disorders such as central sleep apnea (CSA) or obstructive sleep apnea (OSA) or both.[143]

- CSA is characterized by pauses in breathing or shallow breaths during sleep secondary to a lack of respiratory drive, which can last from a few seconds to a few minutes, and can occur multiple times throughout the night, thus disrupting the normal sleep cycle.
- OSA occurs when the airway becomes blocked during sleep, leading to similar pauses in breathing or shallow breathing.[175]

While the sleep disorder may be a result of the brain injury itself, many sleep problems are treatable. Often, the initial step is a thorough review of the individual's sleep habits and routine. It is important to identify if there is a treatable reason for the sleep disorder so that treatment can be initiated and healthier sleep can commence. If the problem is primarily with falling asleep, a simple medication trial may be initiated, such as low-dose melatonin. If the problem is staying asleep, taking a history to identify a cause for the waking (e.g., pain, muscle spasms) may suggest treatment with a muscle relaxant, for instance, or may suggest further evaluation. If the cause of the sleep disorder is another condition, such as enlarged tonsils, surgery may be indicated.

If the waking seems unrelated to any specific reason, a test known as a polysomnogram (a sleep study) may be advised. This test monitors various parameters during sleep, including brain activity, eye movement, heart rate, and oxygen level. The test shows the sleep patterns of the individual, including which part of the sleep cycle is most impacted by the waking. It can also detect seizure activity, which can indicate epilepsy.

Sometimes using oxygen with or without breathing support during sleep may be indicated (see section 3.2).

Sleep medicine specialists are a useful resource to evaluate sleep problems and help to identify solutions.

Sleep? What is that? Levi does not, as a rule, sleep through the night. Some nights he is up only once or twice, but most nights it's four or five times. If he's sick, it can be as many as 10 or more times. This is exhausting for those of us who need to attend to him for repositioning, changing his diaper, entertainment, etc. However, Levi simply does not need the same amount of sleep that a typical person does. We have a few nightly sleep medications that help Levi fall asleep, and a few others for when he cannot stay asleep. His sleep specialist is amazing and has saved our collective sanity.

Levi's father and I divorced when the boys were three. One huge benefit of sharing custody is that the parent who does not have Levi overnight can get some sleep.

However, we recently had a breakthrough. Just before this book was published, Levi had another sleep study to determine why he was not sleeping through the night. Once again, no cause was found. I was frustrated but not surprised. A few weeks later, I noticed that his gums were very swollen where he had had his last few remaining baby teeth (four molars) removed last summer. The permanent molars were breaking through his gums very slowly because he, like many tube-fed children, doesn't chew on anything to help the teeth push through the gums. There were little white blisters where the corners of the permanent molars were going to come through the gum line, and the gum was red and swollen. I wondered if that could be the pain that was keeping him from sleeping. I picked up some oral pain relief gel and put it on the gums that looked sore, and Levi slept through the night! You read that right: He. Slept. Through. The. Night!

What a blessed relief! We had finally found something to help him (and us) get some sleep and get to the root of some of his previously untraceable discomfort. It made so much sense in hindsight; of course his teeth would take longer (months to years instead of weeks) to break through, causing discomfort the whole time. When I followed up with Levi's sleep doctor, he was as surprised as I was that after all these years of struggle and searching for meds that would help him get some sleep, Levi's teeth were at the root of much of his sleep issues. I, however, am just happy to finally have a solution in my cupboard that I can use when Levi isn't sleeping. I am hopeful, too, that sharing this information will provide even one extra night of quality sleep for a family out there like ours.

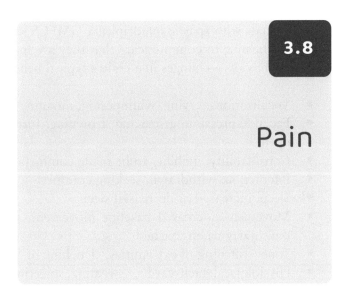

3.8

Pain

It is easier to find men who will volunteer to die, than to find those who are willing to endure pain with patience.

Julius Caesar

Pain was reported in 79 percent of individuals with CP GMFCS levels IV and V,[158] and pain is linked to higher rates of behavioral problems and lower participation.[174] Pain frequency and intensity have also been shown to increase with age in individuals with CP.[160] Children with CP may also have more sensitivity to pain compared to the typical population.[176] The causes of pain can be multiple and may include muscle tone, muscle spasms, uncontrolled movements or body postures, contractures, joint pain, scoliosis, hip displacement, uncomfortable seating, GERD, and constipation. Uncontrolled pain can cause sleep disturbance, which in turn can affect pain tolerance. Hip, thigh, knee, lower leg, feet, and abdomen are the locations of pain most frequently reported by children and adults with CP GMFCS levels IV and V.[160]

Pain may be acute and short lived, intermittent, or chronic. Anxiety or fear of pain may contribute to decreased participation leading to further problems.[176] Early recognition and treatment of pain is important since pain can lead to alterations in sleep, decreased participation, and lower quality of life.[161]

Individuals with spastic quadriplegia GMFCS levels IV and V may not always be able to communicate that they are in pain. Hauer described pain behaviors—changes in a child's typical behavior including:[177]

- Vocalizations: crying, whimpering, moaning
- Facial expression: grimacing, frowning, furrowed brow, eyes wide open
- Consolability: inability to be made comfortable
- Interaction: withdrawn, seeking comfort
- Sleep: increased or decreased sleep
- Movement: increased baseline movement, restless, startles easily, pulls away when touched
- Tone: stiffening of extremities, clenching of fists, back arching
- Physiological: tachycardia,* sweating, shivering, change in color, tears

Assessing pain in individuals who may have communication challenges can be difficult and is best done by parents or close caregivers who know the individual best, and who are therefore the most knowledgeable about when the child or adolescent is in pain. Communicating how they show they are in pain to health care professionals is important, and there are validated pain assessment tools that may be useful for individuals who have communication challenges. These tools typically rely on assessing the individual's facial expressions, movements, activity level, and other pain behaviors noted above. It is important for parents to determine baseline behaviors in order to best determine when a change may indicate pain.

---

* An abnormally rapid heart rate.

We don't always know if Levi is feeling pain. He certainly has different cries, and we recognize his pain cry. We assume that some nights when he is up frequently, he might have pain, so we reposition him and try Tylenol. Levi seems to have sensory differences to some pain as well. For example, he doesn't cry during an IV poke, but he *hates* the blood pressure cuff!

When pain is recognized, the first action should be to find its location, if possible, so that the cause can be determined. At times, the location of the pain may be difficult to pinpoint. Administering over-the-counter analgesics (pain-relieving medication) is often appropriate while searching for the cause and/or location of the pain. Sometimes the location is identified because the pain is present only under certain conditions (e.g., with certain positioning or movements of a limb). Other times the location of the pain is not known and the search for the source is more challenging.

"Occult pain" refers to pain that has an unclear or hidden cause and/or location. Occult pain can arise almost anywhere in the body. Clinicians may begin considering the digestive and urinary systems; other areas to consider include ears and teeth.

Neuropathic pain is a type of chronic pain triggered by the nervous system and may be treated with medication such as gabapentin. If the medication resolves the pain, the diagnosis of neuropathic pain is presumed confirmed.

Individuals with spastic quadriplegia often require medical procedures that themselves may cause pain. This can lead to pain anxiety, which is severe anxiety about the potential of pain. Alleviation of pain anxiety is important.[176] Using distraction, the services of child life specialists, and sedation for painful procedures, when appropriate, are all ways to help alleviate pain anxiety. In some cases, anxiolytic medication (medication prescribed to alleviate symptoms of anxiety disorders) may be helpful during periods of anticipated increased levels of pain; for instance, when an elective surgery is planned with anticipated postoperative pain, or during the recovery and rehabilitation period.

Where pain is perceived to be a significant issue, involving a specialist in pain and palliative care should be considered. Palliative care focuses on improving the quality of life for individuals (children and adults) with serious health conditions and that of their caregivers. It helps to prevent and relieve suffering through addressing pain and other problems, whether physical, psychosocial, or spiritual.[178] Pain and palliative care specialists focus on alleviating pain with a multimodal approach and are expert at considering the role of acute pain sources as well as the role of chronic conditions on exacerbation of pain. They frequently combine nonmedication and medication modalities.

Sensory system

The best and most beautiful things in the world cannot be
seen or even touched. They must be felt with the heart.

Helen Keller

"Sensory" refers to the senses that include vision, hearing, taste, smell, and touch. "Sensation" can be defined as the physical feeling or perception arising from something that happens to or that comes in contact with the body. "Decreased sensation" means a reduction in the ability to perceive sensory stimuli. "Tactile problems" are ones related to the sense of touch. Sensation also includes the ability to sense temperature and pain, where a limb is in space (proprioception), and to identify an object by feeling it (stereognosis).

Hearing

Thirteen percent of children aged five with spastic quadriplegia (all GMFCS levels) have some level of hearing problems, and 5 percent have bilateral deafness.[80] Early screening for hearing loss is needed, and any hearing problems need to be addressed as hearing loss can impact the development of speech, language, and communication (see section 4.2) and cognition (see section 6.2).

Hearing loss can be difficult to evaluate in an individual with cognitive challenges; however, specialized testing is available for those unable to recognize and reliably respond to sounds. For example, the auditory brain stem response (ABR) test uses surface electrodes to measure the brain's reaction to sounds and to show how well the auditory system is working. At some centers, this test can be done without requiring the child to be sedated.

Early referral to an audiologist and a physician specializing in ear, nose, and throat (ENT), also known as an otolaryngologist, as well as a speech and language pathologist is recommended if there is any hearing loss. Regular follow-up will be necessary. Once hearing problems are identified, the needed supports can be identified for the child's maximum participation.

Vision

Thirty-nine percent of children aged five with spastic quadriplegia (all GMFCS levels) have been found to have some level of vision problems, and 16 percent are functionally blind.[80] The prevalence and severity of associated problems have been found to be greater in children at higher GMFCS levels compared with those at lower GMFCS levels.[80] Strabismus, where the eyes do not look in the same direction at the same time, is more common among individuals with CP than in the typical population.[179] (Strabismus is often referred to as having crossed eyes or a squint.) Cerebral (or cortical) visual impairment (CVI), caused by injury in the visual processing areas of the brain, and not related to problems with the eyes themselves, is more common among children with CP.[180]

Early screening for vision problems should be done, and if there are vision concerns, an early referral to a pediatric ophthalmologist is important. A pediatric ophthalmologist is a physician who specializes in childhood onset vision and eye health concerns.* Vision development is rapid from birth to age six, but visual acuity (sharpness) can continue to change throughout life. Regular follow-up will be necessary. As with hearing, once vision problems are identified, it helps determine what supports the child needs for maximum participation.

Sensation

Sensory input gives us much information about the outside world, which we then incorporate into our learning. For instance, if we feel the heat from sitting too close to a fire, we learn to move a comfortable distance away. Similarly, if we feel that we have sticky fingers from having ice cream drip on them, the sensation prompts us to clean our hands. These examples show how sensation allows us to take information from the world, incorporate it into our learning, and finally to choose an action in response to that sensation. When sensation is diminished, the information from the environment is therefore diminished, and the opportunity for using that information for learning and for subsequent action is diminished.

Individuals with spastic quadriplegia often exhibit limited use of the hands despite encouragement, at least in part because their diminished sensation prevents them from obtaining sufficient information about their environment. This creates a chain of circumstances that reduces functional hand use. They may also be extra sensitive to tactile stimulation; for example, certain foods or clothes or being touched by people.[180]

Decreased sensation can also include cold extremities. Ninety-three percent of children with CP GMFCS levels IV and V were reported to have cold extremities.[158] This can affect hands, feet, or both, and for many it can be independent of ambient temperature. Parents often wonder if their child having very cold feet is cause for concern. Although consideration should be given to other reasons for poor circulation, having cold feet is almost never a reason for alarm. The temperature changes do not commonly indicate a problem with circulation that needs treatment

---

* An optometrist can evaluate for some concerns with vision, but they are not trained to do surgery on the eyes.

and are most commonly related to the autonomic nervous system being affected by CP.

Early referral to an occupational and behavioral therapist can help to find ways to incorporate sensory integration techniques, modify the environment, and lessen discomfort.[180]

Levi seems to have some sensory differences, especially when it comes to temperature regulation. He seems to have cold legs and feet, and he can spike a low-grade fever for no apparent reason. That's why we take his temperature in his ear, as readings on his forehead are frequently inaccurate.

Levi's vision was impacted by the same brain damage that caused his CP. He was checked for ROP (retinopathy of prematurity*) prior to the ostomy takedown, and his eyes were normal. But after the ostomy surgery, the doctors could see he had optic nerve atrophy and a cortical vision impairment. We know that he can see somewhat, but we don't know how much. He looks toward sounds (his hearing is not affected), and he seems to visually attend to things that are in his near vision. My best guess is that he would fall under the VFCS level IV. He has a cortical vision impairment† and optic nerve atrophy.‡ He can see up close but not father than about 10 feet. He has more success seeing with adaptations such as larger images, brighter images on a dark background, and images accompanied by sound.

---

* A condition affecting the eyes of premature infants in which problems with the development of the retina can lead to vision problems or blindness.

† A neurological condition where the brain's visual processing centers are damaged, leading to partial or complete loss of vision despite healthy eyes.

‡ Degeneration of the optic nerve, resulting in decreased vision or blindness due to impaired transmission of visual information from the eye to the brain.

Key points Chapter 3

- General health considerations are addressed across individual body systems, but it is important to remember that they are all interconnected.
- Respiratory issues are the most common cause of morbidity or mortality in individuals with CP. Individuals with spastic quadriplegia face a high risk of developing chronic lung conditions. There are a variety of treatments that can help to improve respiratory function and decrease the risk of respiratory illness.
- Individuals with spastic quadriplegia often have challenges with feeding and swallowing, which can give rise to problems with nutrition. When these challenges interfere with safe swallowing or efficient mealtimes, the multidisciplinary team may recommend a feeding tube to supplement nutrition.
- Digestive challenges are common; they can cause pain, impact respiratory health, and contribute to other medical problems. Staying on top of digestive health is important for the overall health and quality of life of the individual with spastic quadriplegia.
- While incontinence is the most common urinary system problem, other problems include the need to urinate frequently and urgently, hesitancy, and urinary retention.
- Epilepsy is common among individuals with spastic quadriplegia. Treatments are available.
- Adequate sleep is necessary for brain development, and the disruption of sleep and sleep deprivation has been shown to have many negative effects. Sleep medicine specialists can help to evaluate sleep problems and identify solutions.
- Pain is common among individuals with spastic quadriplegia who may not always be able to communicate that they are in pain. Involving specialists in pain and palliative care, medical professionals who focus on alleviating pain with a multimodal approach, should be considered.
- Sensory problems can include problems with vision and processing visual input, hearing and processing auditory input, and decreased sensation and a lack of awareness of the position and movement of the body (proprioception).
- Addressing general health issues as comprehensively as possible serves as a foundation allowing individuals to more fully participate in life.

Chapter 4

Developmental progress and maximizing function

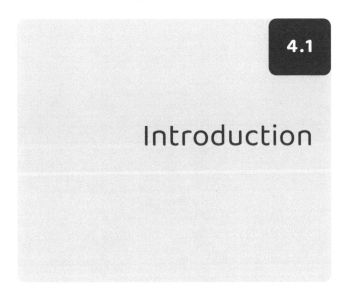

Introduction

The secret of getting ahead is getting started.
Mark Twain

The previous chapter addressed level 1 considerations—general health. This chapter addresses the next level—developmental progress and maximizing function to facilitate participation.

USEFUL WEB RESOURCES

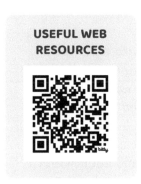

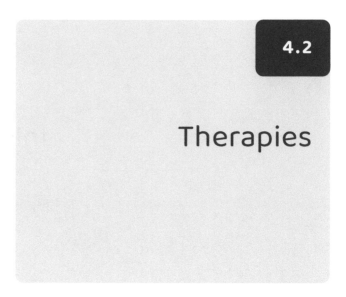

4.2

Therapies

The nice thing about teamwork is that
you always have others on your side.

Margaret Carty

Many children with spastic quadriplegia attend physical therapy, occupational therapy, and/or speech and language pathology at various points during their development. Therapy is defined by Rosenbaum and colleagues as:

> *A process of helping a family (and a child) to learn ways for a child to function optimally in their many environments. It ... involves using the therapist's expertise to explore ways that will enable the child and the family to live as fully and functionally as possible.*[181]

Obviously, this definition extends to the adolescent and adult with CP as well. Improvement in function should be the primary goal of therapy.

This section covers:

- **Physical therapy**
- **Occupational therapy**
- **Speech and language pathology**[*]
- **Delivery of therapy services**
- **Getting the most out of appointments**

Therapists are a vital part of the care team for a child and adolescent with spastic quadriplegia. They not only provide habilitative recommendations for developmental opportunities but also are an additional set of clinical eyes that interact more frequently with the child and family than the medical team (who often only see the individual every few months). Note that "habilitation" refers to the process of *developing* skills and abilities in individuals, while rehabilitation focuses on *restoring* skills and functions in individuals who lost them due to injury, illness, or other factors.

The role of therapy services in supporting the child or adolescent with spastic quadriplegia is to harness any ability they have and maximize their potential for function despite any limitations the brain injury may impose on their progress. However, therapists cannot give the child or adolescent strength or better motor control. If, for example, a child's ability includes some use of their left arm for function, but no use of their right arm or either leg for significant function, they should be encouraged to use the left arm as much as possible to maximize their participation in life. They may have the ability to mobilize themselves independently using a power wheelchair with a left-sided joystick and to use their left hand for fine motor skills and self-care. If their strength is in learning and social interaction, maximizing their ability to participate in such should be a focus as well.

---

* There are other types of therapy offered by specialists: for example, play therapists, music therapists, and recreational therapists. A recreational therapist is qualified to provide recreational therapy services in the US and Canada. There may be an equivalent professional in other countries.

We have used speech therapy, PT, and OT for Levi's entire life. At different times, we have focused more heavily on speech therapy or PT, or gone to assistive technology specialists to try to figure out the best equipment for Levi's ever-changing needs. We do not focus on providing therapy to Levi as his parents, as he has made it clear he does not want us to do that. We do stretches and such, but stander time and eye gaze time is done at school. We revisit this decision fairly often, and if Levi lets us know he wants to try using his devices at home, we will do that.

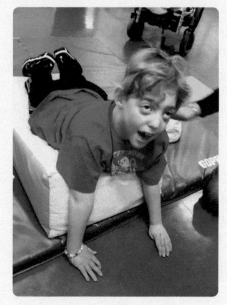

Levi attending physical therapy.

Physical therapy

Physical therapists provide services that develop, maintain, and restore a person's maximum movement and functional ability.[182] Physical therapists have different titles in different countries: in many countries they are called physiotherapists. In this book, we use the terms "physical therapist" and "physical therapy."*

---

* In Ireland, the term "physical therapist" and "physiotherapist" are not interchangeable. There, a physical therapist is someone trained specifically in the manual treatment of soft tissues, mostly massage.

Services that pediatric physical therapists provide for children and adolescents with CP may include:[84]

- Developmental activities
- Movement and mobility
- Strengthening
- Motor learning
- Balance and coordination
- Recreation, play, and leisure
- Daily care activities and routines
- Equipment design, making, and fitting
- Tone management
- Assistive technology (including orthoses)
- Posture, positioning, and lifting

Physical therapists work as part of the multidisciplinary team taking care of the child or adolescent.

Though physical therapists may select treatments designed to improve functional activities, the treatments themselves are often not strictly functional activities. For example, a child's goal may be to be able to assist with stand-pivot transfers.* During the evaluation, the physical therapist may identify limited ankle range of motion (ROM) and weak hip and knee extensors as the underlying problems preventing the child from meeting their goal. As a result, the physical therapist might include casting (to address the limited ROM) and isolated strengthening exercises (to address the weak extensors) in the plan of care for that child. These treatments address the underlying problems, but they themselves are not functional activities. However, as the underlying problems are reduced, the treatment will shift to task-specific functional activities. In this example, the child begins to practice helping more with stand-pivot transfers.

We now address some elements of physical therapy (PT) in more detail.

---

* Moving an individual from one position of sitting to another position of sitting, for example, or from a wheelchair to a bed, using a standing position as a midpoint.

a) Strengthening

Lack of muscle strength is one of the primary problems, but muscle strength is further affected by the development of the secondary problems (abnormal muscle growth and bone development). We saw in section 2.5 that muscle strength was reduced in children with spastic quadriplegia. Historically, strengthening was frowned upon because it was thought to increase spasticity. However, it now is known to increase the force-producing capability, not the spasticity, of the muscle,[183] and therefore strengthening is recommended.

Severe motor problems can make it challenging or impossible to participate in traditional strengthening exercises. The physical therapist can determine which exercises are appropriate for the child based on their motor abilities and developmental stage. Muscles can be strengthened in different positions, and strengthening may be functional. For example, for an individual who is GMFCS level IV, strengthening may include moving from a sitting position to a standing position with assistance. Strengthening may also include weight-bearing activities, especially in young children, to help with muscle growth.

In addition to doing focused muscle strengthening exercises, strengthening has to be built into normal life. For the small child, a variety of positions can provide an opportunity to strengthen the muscles during play. Often, those same positions can be used to achieve both stretch and strength. The need for strengthening also applies to the older child and adolescent.

b) Postural control and balance training

Individuals with spastic quadriplegia may struggle with posture and balance. PT often involves equipment for supported positioning and enhancing balance. For example, the physical therapist may use supported sitting exercises to help improve trunk control, strength, and balance.

Individuals with spastic quadriplegia may also benefit from performing postural control exercises in a therapeutic pool. Children with severe motor problems may be able to move more freely and participate more actively in therapy in water due to the buoyancy it provides.

c) Functional mobility training

Physical therapists specialize in movement, and a significant amount of PT is focused on practicing functional mobility. The physical therapist selects specific mobility activities or tasks based on the individual's age and function, as well as the family's goals.

For individuals with spastic quadriplegia, functional mobility training includes using equipment such as gait trainers, standers, and wheelchairs, addressed further in section 4.4.

For very young children, physical therapists emphasize practicing developmental activities such as rolling or crawling when appropriate to the individual's motor abilities. Later, they may emphasize moving from one position to another, such as transferring using a transfer board.[*] Depending on the child's function and environmental demands, physical therapists may teach children to use compensatory movements[†] or recommend the use of orthoses or mobility aids[‡] to maximize the child's ability to assist in their movement.

For older children, adolescents, and adults, functional mobility training includes how a person moves around in their environment, including transfers and use of mobility aids.

Physical therapists (in collaboration with other members of the multidisciplinary team) are a great source of guidance on mobility aids and orthoses to use in daily life. Specific gait training interventions used during therapy may include treadmill training, partial body weight support treadmill training, and various forms of assisted and even

---

[*] A piece of equipment that facilitates movement between surfaces, such as from a bed to a chair or from a wheelchair to a toilet.

[†] For example, nonreciprocal rather than reciprocal crawling. Reciprocal crawling involves coordinated movements of opposite hands and knees to move forward; nonreciprocal crawling refers to any form of movement (e.g., using a single hand to drag themselves forward without coordinating both sides of the body).

[‡] Mobility aids (also termed "assistive devices," "assistive mobility devices," "walking aids," "mobility aids," and "gait aids") vary in the level of support they provide. Here they are listed in order of least to most support:
  - Canes (walking sticks)
  - Crutches
  - Reverse walker
  - Gait trainer (a device that is more supportive than a walker but less supportive than a wheelchair)
  - Wheelchair

robotic training. The emphasis during these interventions is not only on strengthening and weight-bearing to build bone strength, but also on practicing a high number of repetitions or steps, providing the opportunity to learn from errors, decreasing support, and getting practice in a variety of environments. However, gait training requires a great degree of head and trunk control and ROM that not all individuals with spastic quadriplegia possess.

It is worth noting that standing and gait training are for exercise, bone health, and developing mobility but will not necessarily lead to independent walking. It's important to have fun with these activities while participating with peers or siblings. It is also worth noting that standing is an important skill to achieve and maintain so the person can participate maximally in stand-pivot transfers.

Finally, research shows that powered mobility devices (e.g., ride-on cars, powered wheelchairs) can provide children who have spastic quadriplegia with opportunities for development and participation.[184,185,186] (See Figure 4.2.1.) More information on powered mobility is included in **Useful web resources.**

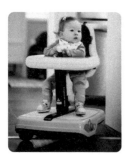 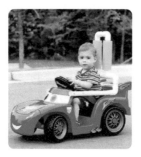 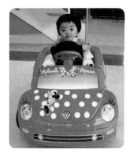

Figure 4.2.1 Permobil Explorer Mini (left). Ride-on cars modified by the Go Baby Go program (middle and right).

d) Stretching

Stretching is not a task-specific functional activity, but it is still important in spastic quadriplegia.

The physical therapist can provide guidance, but stretching must be built into the activities of normal life. We saw in Chapter 2 that two to four hours of stretching per day is required for normal muscle growth, and the typically developing child gets this amount of stretch during the day when they get up and start to move about, run, and play. We also saw that lack of muscle growth leads to contractures in people with spastic quadriplegia.

Stretching is required throughout growth for the young child, the older child, and the adolescent with spastic quadriplegia. How this stretching is achieved may vary over the years, but the need for it remains constant. There are also critical periods when stretching is especially important, which coincide with the periods of most rapid growth: the first three years and during puberty.

Though we refer to stretching muscles, what is actually being stretched is the muscle-tendon unit (MTU) and the associated joint. The methods used for stretching depend on a number of factors, including level of spasticity, muscle tightness, age, and developmental stage.

Traditionally, stretching was done by performing slow *passive* stretching[*] of spastic muscles. However, due to the number of hours of stretching needed to achieve muscle growth and weak evidence supporting the efficacy of passive stretching, greater emphasis is now placed on other, active methods of achieving muscle stretch.[187] Novak and colleagues concur that stretching in isolation appears to be ineffective and do not recommend it since effective substitutes exist.[14] Sometimes passive stretching is still needed but should not be the only method used.

The following describes different methods of stretching (any number of methods may be used simultaneously).

i) Positioning

A variety of positions can be used throughout the day to achieve sustained muscle stretching to promote muscle growth. It is important that the child or adolescent gets a variety of positions throughout the day and does not spend too much time in one position. They may have favorite positions, but it is important to vary them.

---

[*] When another person stretches an individual's muscle.

For individuals with spastic quadriplegia, this positioning may include using a stander to stand upright (see Table 4.4.1) or sitting in various positions with assistance. It may also include prone positioning, which means placing an individual on their stomach. Nighttime positioning can be carried out using orthoses, splints, and special sleep systems. However, given the prevalence of sleep problems in individuals with spastic quadriplegia, if orthoses, splinting, and special positioning at night interfere with sleep, a balance between nighttime stretching and good sleep needs to be found. The benefits and drawbacks of each need to be weighed.

ii) Orthoses

An orthosis (also termed "brace" or "splint") is a device designed to hold specific body parts in position in order to modify their structure and/or function. One of the goals of orthoses is to achieve muscle stretch for a longer duration.

Night splints, such as ankle-foot orthoses (AFOs), which cover the ankle joint and foot, plus knee immobilizers,* may also be used to achieve stretching at night. Wearing an AFO plus a knee immobilizer allows stretching of the calf muscles. Night splints are worn to tolerance during sleep. Wearing one knee immobilizer each night and alternating between right and left may help if wearing both at once is too much.

Orthoses are discussed in section 4.4.

iii) Casting

Casting consists of putting a joint in a plaster of paris or a fiberglass cast (e.g., a below-knee cast to stretch the tight calf muscles). Fiberglass casts are lighter and allow for weight-bearing. Serial casting is the application, removal, and reapplication of stretching casts (e.g., weekly, for four to six weeks) to gain ROM with each subsequent casting until the desired ROM is achieved.

---

* A knee immobilizer consists of a soft knee wrap, rigid aluminum struts, and straps to adjust the fit. As the name suggests, it prevents the knee from moving.

iv) Active movement

Active movement is exactly what it sounds like. Optimally, the child or adolescent should get plenty of active movement through the entire ROM of the joints. Individuals can remove orthoses if they are hindering doing a task and replace them during downtime for a prolonged muscle stretch. This gives them a combination of active movement that may not be in the best position and static stretch in the ideal position.

The approach used in physical therapy and many of the treatments are also used in occupational therapy, addressed next.

Occupational therapy

An occupational therapist uses everyday activities (occupations) to promote health, well-being, and independence throughout an individual's life.[188] Occupational therapists work with children to build confidence and independence in a variety of ways. In order of priority (i.e., if first doesn't work, go to second), these are:

- Completing meaningful tasks to maximize independent movement, strength, and coordination
- Compensating or modifying activities or the environment to enable successful task completion
- Recommending or providing equipment (e.g., orthoses, wheelchairs, bathing equipment), and/or technology that can increase independence when performing activities

For example, if an individual is unable to hold a fork due to spasticity and decreased dexterity, activities might be:

- Using an overnight orthosis for increased ROM, engaging in strengthening, and doing coordination exercises
- Raising the plate and using an adaptive fork
- Using a universal cuff (see section 4.4) to hold the fork

Areas covered in occupational therapy (OT) include, but are not limited to:

- Daily living skills such as dressing, feeding, grooming, and bathing
- Fine motor skills such as writing, using scissors, and manipulating toys

- Cognitive skills such as sticking to a schedule, learning to play a new game, and following step-by-step directions
- Visual motor skills and visual perceptual skills such as using eye movement to explore and interact with the environment
- Participation in the day-to-day activities that motivate the person, such as play, sport, crafts, and vocational skills

Some occupational therapists—certified hand therapists—also specialize in upper limb involvement.

Occupational therapists can be especially important as the child grows, when daily activities and independent living skills become more demanding and potentially more difficult to complete. Below are some areas an occupational therapist may address with individuals who have spastic quadriplegia.

a) Stretching and strengthening

As with physical therapy, occupational therapy contains elements of stretching and strengthening to directly help with an activity. For example, a supported sitting position may be used to improve function and participation in activities that require use of the hands. (See the section on physical therapy above for more details on stretching and strengthening.)

b) Orthoses

Occupational therapists play a large role in assessing and identifying appropriate orthoses to enhance participation in activities of daily living. Orthoses are discussed in more detail in section 4.4.

c) Activities of daily living

Occupational therapy to enhance an individual's ability to perform or assist with activities of daily living (ADLs) is goal based and informed by the individual's gross motor abilities, cognitive abilities, and presence of other problems. For example, occupational therapists often screen for vision problems and use this information to select appropriate treatment activities, considering how those vision problems may impact motor abilities such as hand use.

ADL-related therapy activities also change depending on age:

- Young children: the focus is on activities that feel like play, encouraging the child to engage and participate in play.
- Middle childhood to adolescence: the focus is on increased engagement in family responsibilities, organized activities, and socialization such as typing, writing, or texting for access to social communication.
- Adolescence to young adulthood: the focus is on building skills for living as independently as possible and managing adult tasks such as scheduling appointments or directing care.

ADLs for individuals with spastic quadriplegia of any age focus on the ability to assist with tasks such as dressing, grooming, feeding, bathing, and toileting. For example, this may include working with an individual to put their arm through their shirtsleeves while their caregiver assists with dressing. Occupational therapists can recommend adaptive equipment for completing ADLs, addressed in more detail in section 4.4.

d) Building autonomy

An important part of occupational therapy is building autonomy and maximizing the capacity for the individual to be independent. Goals for independence are set based on functional and cognitive abilities. For individuals with spastic quadriplegia, these goals may center on the ability to direct their caregivers and advocate for themselves in their care. For example, occupational therapists may discuss what appropriate caregiver relationships look like. This could also involve building medication self-management skills, such as being able to communicate what medications the individual takes and when they take them, or having more general medication knowledge such as how many pills they are supposed to take each day. Some occupational therapists specialize in adaptive driving of a motor vehicle and can assist in determining if this is a safe option.

Speech and language pathology

Speech and language pathology (SLP) is also known as speech and language therapy (SLT). Speech and language pathologists/therapists work with children, young people, and adults to support their speech, language, and communication needs as well as feeding and swallowing difficulties.

- **Speech** refers to saying sounds accurately and in the right places in words. Speech is a motor task.
- **Language** refers to the words and symbols we use, and how we use them for communication. Language is a cognitive task.
  - **Receptive language** refers to understanding information from sounds, words, symbols, signs, gestures, and/or movements.
  - **Expressive language** refers to the ability to communicate thoughts, wants, needs, and/or feelings through words, gestures, signs, and/or symbols.

Speech and language pathologists will assess speech, language, and cognitive skills to determine how to improve communication. The child and adolescent may receive SLP at school, in an outpatient clinic, or both. Just as there is overlap between PT and OT, there is overlap between OT and SLP; for example, in the area of executive function work or in feeding work. The speech-language pathologist will work with parents, caregivers, and teachers to identify strategies to encourage and improve the child's communication at home, in school, and with friends as well as during activities to help develop speech and language skills.

SLP may be done individually or in a group. The following are areas of focus:

- **Language skills** allow a child to communicate in their environment, which encourages the development of cognitive skills. A speech-language pathologist will work on cognitive development by improving language comprehension; building vocabulary; improving how to use words, gestures, and pictures to express thoughts, ideas, and feelings; and improving knowledge of how to answer questions. Language comprehension is needed to be able to follow directions, understand the meaning of words, and understand how words go together.
- **Expressive language** allows a person to ask for what they want and need, to comment or provide information, to ask questions or for clarification if they don't understand, to get attention when needed, and to express feelings.

- **Oral motor skills** improve secretion management (drooling, aspiration of secretions*), which helps improve the ability to move and break down food in preparation for swallowing and speech production.
- **Speech production** can include being able to say individual sounds correctly with correct placement of the lips, tongue, and mouth shape, paired with adequate breath support and control of the breath stream. It also includes making the vocal folds (voice box) vibrate for some sounds and not others. Speech production also can include sequencing these sounds to make words and sequencing more than one word to make a sentence that is understood by others.
- **Communication systems** help children who have more difficulty with talking or may only be able to produce a few words. Speech and language therapy will work on strategies to increase communication by using different communication systems. This may include signs or gestures that the child is able to motorically make with some consistency, simple pictures or speech generating devices.
- **Social communication** includes how to take turns, how to partner with others to exchange ideas, thoughts, jokes, and how to greet others. Social communication often impacts a person's ability to make and maintain friendships.
- **Cognitive-communication skills** include memory, attention, problem-solving, and organization. Attention to the environment, to the communication and language of others, and to what is happening in the environment is very important for cognitive development. Executive function includes many cognitive-communication skills that help the individual plan and get things done.
- **Fostering independence** helps the individual communicate their wants and needs, as well as their feelings. This helps them learn to advocate for themselves.
- **Dysphagia (swallowing disorders) therapy** is useful for determining the best treatment for swallowing dysfunction. Frequently it is recommended that the individual have an instrumental swallow evaluation. This is done either by a videofluoroscopic swallowing study (also called a modified barium swallow study) or a FEES (fiberoptic endoscopic evaluation of swallowing). These studies allow therapists to visualize the coordination of the three phases of feeding and swallowing—the functioning and movement of

---

* Drooling is excess saliva dropping uncontrollably from the mouth. Aspiration is food or liquid entering the airway or lungs instead of the esophagus.

different structures for moving food to the stomach and for protecting the airway. They also determine if there is aspiration of any food or liquids, or if the individual is at risk for aspiration or choking. They can also be useful in providing information on which strategies—positioning, modifying foods, pacing, swallow techniques—may improve swallow safety and function, and determine if the muscles of swallowing are strong enough for more difficult foods or if they get tired quickly.

> We believe that Levi has pretty typical receptive communication.* He has a long processing time, but he can smile in response to a yes/no question. We have tried many types of adaptive communication devices. He has had success with buttons and switches and partial success using a Tobii eye gaze device.† He does not have enough intentional control over fine motor movements, so a touch screen is not helpful. The eye gaze device is the most beneficial, but it tires him quickly, and we are not sure how accurate his vision is with it. He practices using his device during speech time at school.

Delivery of therapy services

Given that the delivery of therapy services is so variable, only some broad points are addressed here. Having a lifelong condition such as spastic quadriplegia does not mean a person will need lifelong, nonstop PT (or other therapies) or, as it is sometimes referred to, the "once a week for life" model.

Guidelines have been developed for determining the frequency of PT and OT services in a pediatric medical setting.[189] The guidelines are based on:

---

* The terms "receptive communication" and "receptive language" are sometimes used interchangeably.

† A system that relies on eye movements to move a cursor on a screen to select messages or symbols to relay communication needs; generally beneficial for individuals with very limited motor movement.

- The child's ability to benefit from and participate in therapy
- The parent's ability to participate in therapy sessions and follow through with activities at home
- The family's decision related to available resources (e.g., time commitment, financial resources)

Four levels of frequency of therapy are identified in the guidelines:[189]

- **Intensive:** More than three times per week—for children who are in an extremely critical period for acquiring a skill or are regressing.
- **Weekly/bimonthly:** One to two times a week to every other week—for children who need frequent therapy and are making continuous progress toward their goals.
- **Periodic:** Once a month or less—best suited to children whose rates of progress are very slow but who require the skilled services of a therapist to periodically assess a home program and adapt it.
- **Consultative:** As needed—best suited for children who have been discharged from therapy, but who benefit from intermittent evaluation by a therapist.

The episodes of care (EOC) model is used for service delivery. An EOC is a period of therapy at the recommended frequency, such as listed above, followed by a therapy break. Ideally, after an EOC, the child generalizes the skills gained in therapy at home, in school, and in the community. For each EOC, the family and therapist work together to set goals, typically no more than two long-term and four short-term goals. Note that referring to "therapy breaks" might sound like getting therapy is the normal state of affairs for a person with CP, but living life, *not* receiving therapy, should be considered the normal state of affairs.

Figure 4.2.2 shows periods when different therapies may be used, interspersed with breaks in therapy, during childhood and adolescence.[190]

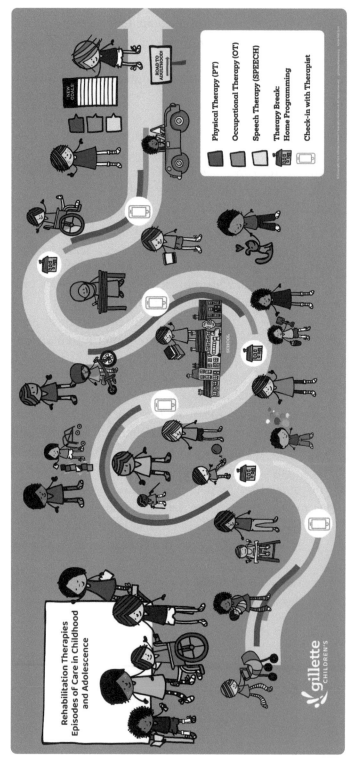

Figure 4.2.2 Episodes of care in childhood and adolescence.[190]

In addition to having formal goals, it is very important that therapists use objective measurement tools to evaluate whether therapy goals have been met. The home program, which includes practicing what the child has learned in therapy at home and incorporating it into normal life, is addressed in section 4.3.

The following are included in **Useful web resources:**

- Cincinnati Children's *Guidelines for Determining Frequency of Therapy* information leaflet for families
- Gillette Children's *Rehabilitation Therapies Episodes of Care in Childhood and Adolescence* information leaflet for families

When Levi was young, we had him in as much therapy as we could. He had private PT, OT, and speech therapy weekly, as well as school-based PT, OT, and speech services weekly. We also tried to do therapy at home (stander, gait training, etc.) as much as possible. I soon realized that Levi was not enjoying doing therapy at home; he would fuss and cry when we made him. By the time he was about eight, he was routinely crying, screaming, or sleeping through therapy sessions, and the therapists could no longer prove that he was making progress. I was frustrated that Levi was not participating in sessions, but I also understood that this was his way of making his wants known. We ended private therapy when we could see that no amount of PT was going to allow him to walk, and no amount of practice with his AAC device would make it easy enough for him to use it to communicate. For our family, we felt that Levi's daily health and happiness was the most important thing for us to focus on, and so we left the therapy to be worked on at school.

Getting the most out of appointments

Life with a diagnosis of spastic quadriplegia involves many appointments, particularly in the early years. During the COVID pandemic, virtual appointments became a feature of health care delivery, and a mixture of in-person and virtual care delivery has remained in place since. Being able to group appointments helps minimize time lost from school and work.

Try to ensure you are getting as much as possible from these appointments. It is useful to go to appointments with a written list of questions and to take notes after each appointment, including what you learned and what is needed to be done next. While portals to access personal medical records (where they exist) have helped reduce the need for taking notes, you may still find it useful to do some note-taking.

To get the most out of appointments on a practical level, try to ensure your child is not tired or hungry. (For that matter, make sure you are not tired or hungry either!)

You know your child best, and to best support their success in therapies, you should engage with the therapy team whenever you have questions, as you might see something they do not. It is also okay to request a break or a change in activity, or to ask about the purpose of an exercise. Partner with your therapists to help to optimize the care being provided.

Nurture the relationship with the professionals treating your child—they are your allies. You may be angry about aspects of your child's diagnosis or treatment, but avoid putting professionals on the receiving end of any misplaced anger. The expression "Don't shoot the messenger" comes to mind. You might be dissatisfied with the range of services provided to your child, for example, but remember that frontline staff are rarely the policy-makers—indeed, they may in fact agree with you. The best management of the condition is achieved when parent and child work together in partnership with the medical professionals.

Good communication between disciplines is also vital for the functioning of the multidisciplinary team. The parent and child are the constants in this relationship; thus, the parent can help support communication between the different team members. No matter how good services are, things can go wrong: for example, a referral might be forgotten, and an appointment might not get scheduled. Supporting communication between team members is particularly important when the child is getting a large part of their care in the community but has to travel to a specialist center from time to time. The parent can play an important role in the smooth coordination of care, so it is helpful to stay organized and keep medical reports together and at hand. This coordinator role may later fall to the adolescent themselves, in time, if their development permits.

Finally, sometimes a particular medical professional is not the right match for the family. If this occurs, be sure to communicate this and try to seek an alternative to optimize the chances of success for the child or adolescent with CP.

I'm a teacher, so I try to schedule all our yearly appointments in the summer. I appreciate the virtual care options that are available, as they are super convenient. At times, keeping track of the number of appointments and names and responsibilities of all the specialists can be overwhelming. More than once I have shown up for an appointment, not having any idea what the appointment was for!

The home program

Exercise is medicine
Susruta

Novak and colleagues defined the home program as the "therapeutic*
practice of goal-based tasks by the child, led by the parent, and supported by the therapist in the home environment."[191] In this book, we
have termed this the "homework" prescribed by therapists.

Practicing what is learned in therapy is very important, but there are
periods when the child or adolescent is not attending therapy in an
episode of care, so it makes sense to have a broader view of the home
program to include all the elements that families do at home to help
manage the condition. These are things that have to become part of life
for the child and adolescent with spastic quadriplegia, such as stretching, strengthening, and wearing orthoses (when prescribed).

The term "home environment" is a collective of the actual home,
school, and wherever the child spends their time. The best people to help

---

* Recommended for reasons of health.

with the child's program are those who regularly interact with the child. In addition to parents, they may be caregivers, siblings, teachers, teaching assistants, grandparents, and childcare providers. They are the optimal ones to provide developmentally appropriate opportunities. Therapists are there to teach, guide, and support.

The saying "It takes a village to raise a child" emphasizes the idea that raising a child, particularly a child with a disability, is not a task that should be shouldered by parents alone. By enlisting the support of others, parents can lighten their load and create a network of individuals who are invested in the child's well-being.

Within the broader view of the home program, it is important to never forget to have fun—one of the F-words introduced in Chapter 1. This section addresses:

- **The homework prescribed by therapists**
- **Postural management**
- **Exercise and physical activity**

We are blessed to have an extensive support system of extended family. Levi's grandmother and aunt are primary caretakers along with his father, his bonus father (stepfather), and me. My sister, Levi's aunt, was a lawyer when my twins were born. She spent so much time in the NICU with them that she went back to school to become a nurse on the cardiovascular intensive care unit at the hospital where the boys were born. My mother was trained as a nurse as well and was Cam and Levi's daily caregiver while I was at work until the boys were five years old.

Having a partner who is hands on in the care of a child with special needs is crucial. Having a child with special needs is stressful, and there are times when it is scary, frustrating, and seemingly impossible. If you have a partner to share the sleepless nights, stress, frustration, and frequent hospital stays with, the impossible is made possible again. Whenever Levi is sick or in the hospital, our extended support system makes a difficult time quite a bit easier.

The homework prescribed by therapists

The benefit of any therapy (PT, OT, SLP/SLT) is only partly gained in the therapy session itself. The real benefits come from regular practice at home.

Families depend on therapists to prescribe evidence-based treatments. Therapists depend on the child or adolescent, with the support of the parent and their network, to get in the practice at home. This is a collaborative relationship. Much of what is learned in therapy has to become part of everyday life for the child or adolescent with spastic quadriplegia in order to be effective.

Working with a therapist is a partnership, and the parent and child or adolescent are partners with the therapist in the decision-making process. It is important that the parent and child or adolescent share with the therapist their goals and what may be less important to them to enable focus on what is truly valued by the team. It is recommended that you talk with your therapist and make sure you have a good under-standing of the activities you'll be carrying out at home and that it is a realistic plan.

When Levi was young, we did many therapeutic activities with him at home. He had a stander, gait trainer, and many seating options. As he has grown, his ability to stand and take steps has faded. He tolerates the stander when he's at school and uses it daily there. We do not do the stander at home as it takes a lot to move it between school and home, and to get him into and out of it. His past two summers have been full of surgery recovery, so standing has not been an option at home.

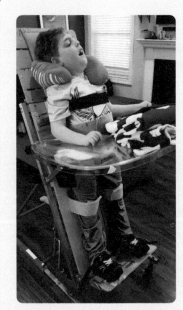

Levi in his stander.

Postural management

Postural management is another constant in the life of the child and adolescent with spastic quadriplegia. "Posture" refers to the position in which a person holds their body while sitting, standing, or lying down. Good posture applies to everyone, not just individuals with CP.

For example, to maintain good posture, a person needs to have adequate strength in their trunk-stabilizing muscles and good balance reactions. This is why the typically developing child cannot sit independently until they are approximately six months old. Individuals with spastic quadriplegia are likely to have some challenges with posture. Due to their musculoskeletal differences, if they cannot optimally support their posture independently, it is important to have support with assistive technology (e.g., adaptive or customized seating) to prevent pain, musculoskeletal changes, and asymmetries insofar as possible. Table 4.3.1 lists recommendations on good posture in sitting, standing, and sleeping. The aim of postural management is to achieve this positioning insofar as possible. Information on postural support systems is included in section 4.4.

Table 4.3.1 Good posture in sitting, standing, and sleeping

GOOD POSTURE IN:	ILLUSTRATION
Sitting • Feet flat on the floor, with hips, knees, and ankles at 90 degrees and both sides of the trunk straight and symmetrical. (If feet cannot reach the floor, something firm, such as a box or book, can be placed under them to ensure they are flat and that the 90-degree angle is achieved.) • Support provided at the sides, if necessary, to ensure the trunk is straight and symmetrical. • Arms close to the body and relaxed. • Head balanced on the neck (not tilted forward or backward).	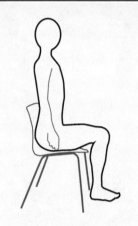
Standing • Feet flat on the floor. • Knees neither locked nor bent. • Abdominal muscles tight and buttocks tucked in. • Shoulders back and down slightly, even, and relaxed. • Head facing forward, not tilted to one side or the other. • Chin tucked and ears over the shoulders.	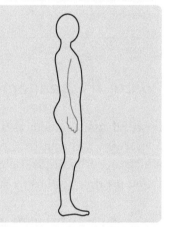
Sleeping • Posture is midline and symmetrical (i.e., the two sides are equal). • Sleeping in a supine position (on the back) is recommended. • If lying on one side, it can be helpful to place a pillow between the legs to keep the spine in good alignment. A pillow under the top arm can also be useful to support good alignment—often the top arm is pulled down by gravity, which can result in curving of the spine or rolling to prone position (sleeping on the front) in the night.	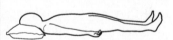

Exercise and physical activity

Verschuren and colleagues published a set of exercise and physical activity recommendations for people with CP under the following headings:[192]

- Cardiorespiratory (aerobic) exercise
- Resistance (muscle strengthening) exercise
- Daily moderate to vigorous physical activity
- Avoiding sedentary behavior (i.e., not being physically inactive)

However, for individuals with spastic quadriplegia, it may not be possible to meet the optimal recommendation of 60 minutes of daily moderate to vigorous physical activity. Even children GMFCS levels I to III have a hard time meeting these guidelines.[193] Knowing that, Verschuren and colleagues recommend focusing on reducing sedentary behavior whenever possible.[192] For people who spend a large part of their day sitting in a wheelchair, even small volumes of light activity, such as supported standing or unsupported sitting out of their wheelchair, may lead to profound health gains.[192]

Adapting the daily routine to include different positions, such as having the individual use a stander, stand in a gait trainer, lie on their tummy propped up on elbows, sit on the edge of the couch, or kneel at the coffee table, can result in an increase in daily physical activity. Specific activities throughout the day, such as eating, brushing teeth, doing homework, watching television, or playing a game, can be associated with a specific, more active position than sitting in a wheelchair. Each of these positions creates demands on different muscles and results in the body having to work harder compared with sitting in a wheelchair where muscles are typically relaxed and not actively using energy.

Creating changes to the daily routine to incorporate activity is the most feasible method for families with busy schedules. Research shows that individuals with CP GMFCS levels IV and V are capable of taking part in community-based physical activity interventions in addition to these home routines without post-exercise pain, fatigue, or serious adverse events.[194] Some of the physical activities that have been successful include riding an adaptive or recumbent bicycle, using an arm or rowing

	GMFCS I 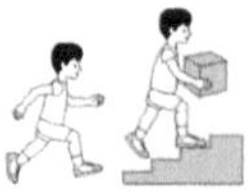	GMFCS II 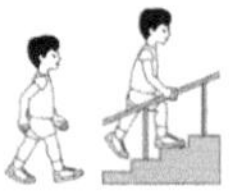
Athletics	Ambulant Athletics – Track and Field	Ambulant Athletics - Track and Field
Swimming	Unaided swimming	Unaided swimming
Football	CP 7-a-side Football	CP 7-a-side Football
Racquet Sports	Standing Badminton Standing Table-Tennis Standing Cricket	Standing Badminton Standing Table-Tennis Standing Cricket Wheelchair Tennis
Individual Sports	Taekwondo Para-Cycling (2/3 wheeler) Para Triathlon Equestrian CP Bowls Standing Archery standing Golf Para Shooting Powerlifting Seated Fencing	Taekwondo Para-Cycling (2/3 wheeler) Para Triathlon Equestrian CP Bowls Standing Archery standing Golf Para Shooting Powerlifting Seated Fencing
Team Sports	Sitting Volleyball Beach ParaVolley Ambulant CP rugby Ambulant Netball	Sitting Volleyball Beach ParaVolley Ambulant CP rugby Ambulant Netball
Winter Sports	Standing Alpine Skiing Standing Nordic Skiing Snowboarding Para Ice Hockey	Standing Alpine Skiing Standing Nordic Skiing Snowboarding Para Ice Hockey
Water Sports	Rowing Sailing Canoeing	Rowing Sailing Canoeing

Figure 4.3.1 Sports and para sports for individuals with CP across the GMFCS levels. Reproduced with kind permissions from World Abilitysport. GMFCS illustrations Version 2 © Bill Reid, Kate Willoughby, Adrienne Harvey, and Kerr Graham, The Royal Children's Hospital Melbourne.

GMFCS III	GMFCS IV	GMFCS V
RaceRunning Seated Athletics - Track and Field	RaceRunning Seated Athletics - Track and Field	RaceRunning Seated Athletics – Track and Field
Unaided swimming		
Frame Football	Frame Football Powerchair Football	Powerchair Football
Wheelchair Badminton Wheelchair Tennis Seated Table Tennis Wheelchair Cricket	Wheelchair Badminton Wheelchair Tennis Seated Table Tennis Table Cricket	Table Cricket
Para-Cycling (2/3 wheeler) Seated Fencing Para Triathlon Boccia Equestrian CP Bowls Seated Archery seated Wheelchair Slalom Para Shooting Powerlifting	Para-Cycling (2/3 wheeler) Seated Fencing Boccia CP Bowls Seated Archery seated Para Shooting Powerlifting Trap Driving Wheelchair Slalom	Wheelchair Slalom Boccia Para Shooting Trap Driving
Sitting Volleyball Wheelchair Basketball Wheelchair Rugby	Sitting Volleyball Wheelchair Basketball Wheelchair Rugby	
Sitting Alpine Skiing Standing/Sitting Nordic Skiing Wheelchair Curling Para Ice Hockey	Sitting Nordic Skiing Wheelchair Curling	
Rowing Sailing Canoeing	Sailing Canoeing	Assisted Sailing

ergometer,* swimming, wheelchair dancing, and using free weights, exercise bands, or a weight machine. Therapists can guide individuals to find an adapted community program that is of interest and is able to meet their physical needs. The community-based environment may provide additional benefits of socialization and increased motivation that can lead to further improvements in quality of life.

It is important to remember that increasing activity in any way possible, even small position changes throughout the day, may have great health benefits; therefore, they should be started small and increased as able. Some individuals with spastic quadriplegia, however, may wish to take part in more active forms of exercise.

World Abilitysport, an international organization for the development of para sports,† has developed a list of sports suitable for CP at all GMFCS levels. See Figure 4.3.1.

The Peter Harrison Centre for Disability Sport at Loughborough University in the UK has published two excellent guides specifically for people of all ages with CP. The first, *Fit for Life*, is for people with CP who are new to exercise. The second, *Fit for Sport*, is for people who want to take their athletics to a more advanced level. The first guide contains a very useful table, "What type of exercise can I do?" listing advantages and disadvantages with adaptations and advice for each type of exercise. Both guides are included in **Useful web resources.**

An appointment with a physical therapist, occupational therapist, or a recreational therapist is useful if people need further guidance on how to create an exercise program that suits their needs and abilities. The next section on assistive technology includes adaptive recreational equipment, which helps to make participation in various recreational or leisure pursuits possible or just even easier.

Finally, the special needs of an individual with spastic quadriplegia can be a challenge on family finances. It is worth checking out all possible sources of funding, as there may be more possibilities than first realized.

---

* A stationary exercise machine that simulates rowing or arm cycling.

† Competitive sports specifically designed or adapted for individuals with physical, sensory, or intellectual disability.

Assistive technology

Determine that the thing can and shall be done,
and then we shall find the way.

Abraham Lincoln

"Assistive technology"[*] refers to products and services designed to enhance the functional capabilities and independence of individuals with disabilities to allow them to participate.[195] This section addresses the following assistive technology commonly used by individuals with spastic quadriplegia:

- Seating, standing, and mobility aids
- Adaptive beds and sleep systems
- Adaptive equipment for activities of daily living
- Augmentative and alternative communication
- Environmental control devices
- Orthoses
- Adaptive recreational equipment

---

[*] In the US, some assistive technology is referred to as "durable medical equipment" (DME) for medical insurance purposes.

It is important to note that this is not an exhaustive list, and that assistive technology continues to improve and develop.

Assistive technology should be selected based on assessments performed by a multidisciplinary team including professionals (e.g., physician, physical and occupational therapists, speech-language pathologist, orthotist) in conjunction with the individual and their family. An individual's unique health needs and the family's care and function goals help guide what assistive technology is best suited for the individual. The family knows the individual best and their own particular home and circumstances. In some cases, it is worth doing some reading to be as informed as possible to help choose the most appropriate assistive technology. Regular reevaluation is important, the frequency of which depends on the individual and the product.

Some pointers on making your home more accessible are included in **Useful web resources.**

Seating, standing, and mobility aids

Seating, standing, and mobility aids provide improved function during sitting, standing, and movement. Individuals with spastic quadriplegia GMFCS levels IV and V often have high equipment needs for these functions. The following are commonly used by individuals with spastic quadriplegia:

a) **Floor sitters**
b) **Adaptive chairs**
c) **Standers**
d) **Gait trainers**
e) **Adaptive strollers**
f) **Wheelchairs**
g) **Transfer aids**
h) **Vehicle transportation**

a) Floor sitters

Young children do a lot of playing and learning at floor level. Floor sitters provide postural support for the child with spastic quadriplegia who cannot independently sit. They allow the child to sit and therefore interact and play at floor level with other children.

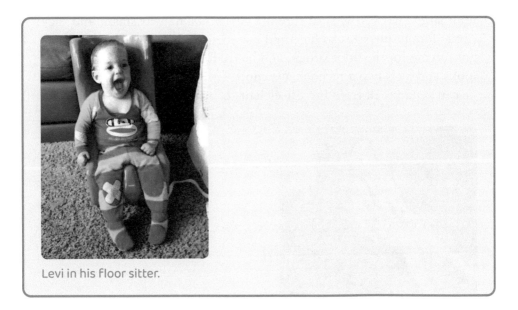

Levi in his floor sitter.

b) Adaptive chairs

Adaptive chairs provide a supported seating option for children with spastic quadriplegia. They may be useful when alternative seated positioning is needed at home or in school (see Figure 4.4.1).

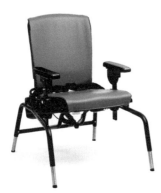

Figure 4.4.1 Adaptive chair. Reproduced with kind permission from Rifton Equipment.

Levi has used or trialed almost every type of adaptive equipment on the market. When he was small, he had multiple types of floor sitters. One had a base with wheels so he could be pushed around the house. These floor sitters worked well to support Levi while he was small, and they came in multiple sizes so he could use them as he grew. Eventually he got too big for the floor sitters, and he trialed a Chill-Out Chair, which looks and feels like a recliner. We choose to keep his chair at school so he can get a break from his wheelchair throughout the schoolday.

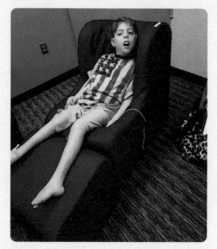

Levi in his Chill-Out Chair.

c) Standers

Standers are devices that allow for the best possible upright standing position for prolonged weight-bearing.[196] Individuals with spastic quadriplegia often face challenges with independent standing. A delay in the ability or inability to stand independently can lead to an increased risk of osteopenia, hip subluxation, and lower extremity contractures. Limited standing is also associated with pain and challenges with respiratory health and digestive function.[197]

There are many types of standers, detailed in Table 4.4.1. As with all equipment, choosing the most appropriate takes careful evaluation. A systematic review found that standing programs positively impact bone density; hip stability; range of motion (ROM) in the hips, knees, and ankles; and spasticity.[198]

Table 4.4.1 Standers

TYPE	EXPLANATION	IMAGE
Supine stander	The individual is placed in a supine position (on their back), then tilted into an upright position. Straps can be placed around the knees, pelvis, and chest for support. In the upright position, the stander is slightly tilted back. Supine standers can be suitable for individuals who struggle with head control, as the tilt allows gravity to keep the head upright and can sometimes slowly help the individual improve their control. An added tray can provide support for the upper extremities and allow the individual to do activities.	Two supine standers; the second version shows a stander both with a tray (middle image) and without a tray (bottom image).

Cont'd.

TYPE	EXPLANATION	IMAGE
Prone stander	The individual is placed in a prone position (on their stomach), then tilted into an upright position. These standers are typically most appropriate for individuals who do not have scoliosis and display good head control. An added tray can provide support for the upper extremities and allow the individual to do activities.	
Multiposition stander	The individual can be placed in a supine, prone, or upright position. The stander can convert between supine and prone positioning, with a removable headrest and adjustable foot supports, support pads, and tray table supports. These standers may be well suited for individuals whose head control varies greatly or who would benefit from having multiple positioning options.	Multiposition stander in supine position (top image) and prone position (bottom image).

Cont'd.

TYPE	EXPLANATION	IMAGE
Sit-to-stand stander	The individual can change from a seated position to a standing position with this stander. It allows for an easy transition between activities that require both positions and may be especially helpful in school. It also allows lateral transfers out of the stander (from a seated position) as opposed to a dependent lift from the standing position. It is typically appropriate for individuals who have at least fair head control.	
Mobile stander	The individual is typically in an upright position with the support surface at the front of the body. Similar to a wheelchair, the mobile stander has large wheels that can be used to move it. Because it takes up a lot of space, it is not typically used at home, but instead in an adaptive, clinic, or school setting.	

Adapted from Ward and colleagues.[197]

d) Gait trainers

A gait trainer is similar to a walker but offers increased postural support, weight-bearing capabilities, and mobility assistance while walking. Gait trainers typically consist of a wheeled frame with weight-bearing support straps and upper extremity supports such as a tray, handle, or handrail. See Figure 4.4.2.

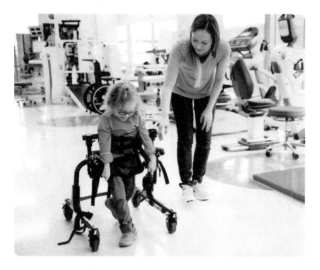

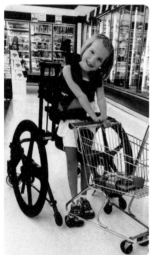

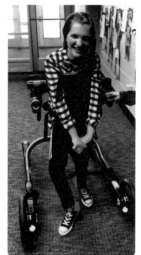

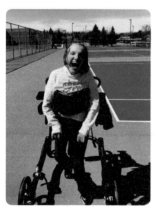

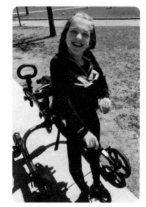

Figure 4.4.2 Gait trainers.

Gait trainers can be used to develop or improve an individual's walking ability, but are often used for exercise. Walking with a gait trainer provides the benefits of improved strength, ROM, self-esteem, participation, and bowel and bladder function.[197]

Given the level of postural support, gait trainers are appropriate for individuals who are incapable of walking unsupported.[197] The gait trainer can be customized to suit an individual's functional ability and needs. For example, additional trunk support can be built into the trainer for those who need it.

e) Adaptive strollers

Adaptive strollers (also known as medical strollers) are tailored to the unique postural, functional, and comfort needs of the individual. Adaptive strollers do not provide independent mobility; instead they are dependent on the parent or caregiver to be moved.

An adaptive stroller may be appropriate for a small child (typically age three to four) or for a child and family without safe access to wheelchair home use and wheelchair transportation. Typically, as the child grows, they will require larger equipment with more sitting support. Once children transition to elementary school, families are encouraged to explore a wheelchair that offers greater mobility independence and/or optimized positioning and pressure-reducing components for the following reasons:

- Increased sitting support and overall stability of the equipment
- Ability for the child to develop independent mobility
- More socially appropriate for children at this age, given that strollers may be more closely associated with an infant or small child
- Easier to participate in transfers (for those who are able)

For these reasons, it is important to consider the individual and caretaker needs, and environmental accessibility, when determining if a wheelchair or stroller is best even for the child's first mobility device. The equipment needs to last several years, and a wheelchair can sometimes offer more room for growth and feature options.

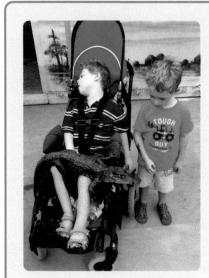

Levi in his adaptive stroller.

f) Wheelchairs

Wheelchairs are designed to allow mobility for an individual who has limited or no ability to walk. They consist of two main parts: the seating system and the mobility base. The aim is to optimize the seating position while maximizing independent mobility. Growing research demonstrates a relationship between independent mobility of any means and cognitive and social development.[197]

There are many types of wheelchairs with a variety of base frame types and styles, seating components, wheel types, and accessories for additional medical supplies and other needs.[196] As the child grows and their positioning and functional needs change, it is important for the multidisciplinary team to continually reevaluate the individual's needs. Common types of wheelchairs are listed in Table 4.4.2.

Table 4.4.2 Wheelchairs

TYPE	DESCRIPTION	IMAGE
Manual wheelchair	A manual wheelchair is self-propelled by the individual or pushed by a caregiver. Thus, independent mobility with a manual wheelchair requires a degree of upper extremity motor control and strength.	 Self-propelled manual wheelchairs (moved by the user) above. Attendant-propelled manual wheelchair (moved by a caregiver) below.

Cont'd.

TYPE	DESCRIPTION	IMAGE
Power-assist wheelchair	A power-assist wheelchair (also known as a power-assisted wheelchair or a power add-on) is designed to enhance the manual propulsion of a standard wheelchair. It provides an extra power boost to the user's manual efforts, making it easier to propel the wheelchair over various terrains or inclines, to protect against shoulder overuse injuries, and to extend the propulsion distance the person can cover. The power-assist feature is typically incorporated into the wheels either as an integrated system or as an attachable device.	
Tilt-in-space (TIS) wheelchair	With a TIS wheelchair, either manual or power, the seat can be tilted back while keeping the seat-to-back angle the same. This feature can help individuals with poor trunk or head control to gain balance and stability. The tilt can be adjusted to increase or decrease the amount of postural support or redistribute pressure while sitting. Use of the tilt feature can also help prepare for safe transfers and with positioning following transfers.	Power TIS wheelchair in TIS position.
Power wheelchair	A power wheelchair (also known as an electric wheelchair or motorized wheelchair) is powered by an electric motor that is controlled by an electronic control system (joystick, buttons, or other devices). It is suitable for individuals with limited upper extremity motor control and strength. It is worth noting that a power wheelchair is a heavy machine and cannot be lifted like a manual wheelchair. Power wheelchairs can have additional features, such as an elevator mechanism enabling the individual to sit comfortably at higher counters. They can allow individuals to stand when and where they want, eliminating the need to transfer to a separate standing device.	

g) Transfer aids

A transfer aid is a form of specialized equipment used to safely transfer an individual from one place to another; for example, moving from their bed to their wheelchair. As children grow, these transfers can become increasingly physically challenging, putting the person assisting and the individual transferring at higher risk of injury. Parents of children who need assistance for transfers have a higher incidence of low back pain than parents of children who can transfer independently.[197] Specialized equipment may help ease the physical challenge of transfers for parents while enabling the child to safely transfer between settings. Common transfer aids include but are not limited to:

- **Manual hydraulic lift:** A freestanding device with a manually operated pump that assists with transfers of the individual in an attached sling. The caregiver operates the pump to raise and lower the individual. The lift has wheels that allow the individual to be moved to the desired location.
- **Electric lift:** A freestanding electrically operated lift. By pressing buttons or switches, the individual in the attached sling is raised and lowered. As with the manual lift, it has wheels that allow the individual to be moved to the desired location.
- **Ceiling lift:** A ceiling-mounted motorized system with ceiling tracks for movement to desired locations in the home. It operates similar to a freestanding lift, with a sling for transport and a remote control for moving the individual to the desired location. See Figure 4.4.3.

While useful in some situations, lifts do have limitations and they will not work everywhere in the home. For instance, they do not allow for transferring into a bathtub or onto a couch unless there is enough space beneath it for the base of the lift to fit. Ceiling lifts are also limited to the spaces in the home where ceiling tracks are installed.

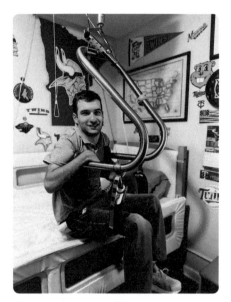 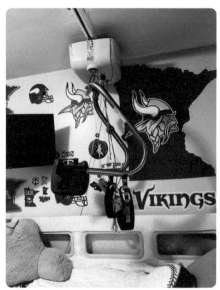

Figure 4.4.3 Ceiling lift.

h) Vehicle transportation

As children get older, they eventually outgrow commercial child car and booster seats, which then need to be replaced by specialized equipment to provide adequate safety and postural support. Medical car seats are specialized for this purpose and can accommodate more weight than commercial car seats can.

Transportation should be considered from an early stage as it is difficult to lift an older child into a car seat. In addition, a wheelchair may be too heavy or not possible to fold to put in the trunk. Wheelchair accessible vehicles are specifically designed to accommodate wheelchairs. These vehicles feature a lowered floor or ramp for easy wheelchair entry and exit, wheelchair tie-downs to secure the wheelchair in place, and a vehicle-mounted seat belt to ensure safety for the wheelchair user during transport.

When Levi was an infant and a small child, he could stand with assistance and make a walking motion with his legs, though he couldn't sit up or stand under his own power. As an infant, he could use a normal twin stroller and car seat. As a toddler, he used an adaptive stroller, and when he was about three or four, he received his first manual wheelchair. It was at this time that we went through the process of getting our first modified minivan. We knew by then that Levi would likely always need a mobility aid and that having a modified van would make life easier.

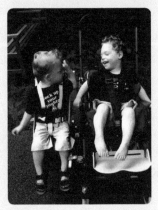

Cam beside Levi in his adaptive stroller.

When you have a child who uses a wheelchair, you realize quickly that the wheelchair will need to be updated frequently. As the child grows, the wheelchair can expand and be made a bit bigger so it can last a few years. Often it will need minor tweaks and changes to the seating, headrest, footrest, wheels, seating system, chest strap, etc. There are so many options for personalization and modification, and an assistive technology specialist can help guide the changes. We generally do a seating modification once or twice a year and a full seating evaluation every two years. We are an active family, so for us the wheelchair needs to be rugged enough to go on hikes and be pushed through the snow and sand.

As a young child, Levi used a supine stander, and as he grew, he got a multipositional stander. We have always kept the stander at his school, and that is where Levi does his standing. Levi doesn't really enjoy standing because it's hard work for him. But he tolerates it well, and the benefits outweigh his slight discomfort. As long as he has his shows to listen to, he will stand for up to an hour a day.

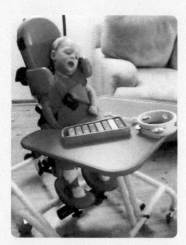

Levi in his stander.

When Levi was about 12 years old and 75 lb, we put a ceiling lift into his bedroom and bathroom. We use this lift to help us give him baths safely. The lift has a bath sling that holds Levi and allows us to safely bring him from his bed to his bathtub and back again. It is a huge help for us!

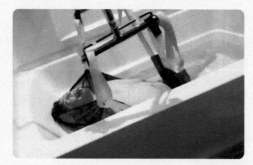

Levi bathing.

Getting a modified vehicle is a big process that takes many months. We do a ton of driving and replace our modified vehicles about every five or six years or 200,000 miles. For us, our county waiver (state medical assistance plan) helps pay for modifying the vehicle, and we get a loan for the base cost. We are lucky in Minnesota to have a few mobility specialist van dealers. It's important to go to each dealership and evaluate the physical modification to see if it is the right fit for you. There are rear-entry, side-entry, and even front-entry vans/SUVs. Some ramps fold out manually while others are automatic. Some ramps are great for the snow, and others not so much. This past fall we bought a handicap-accessible Chevrolet Traverse, and it is perfect for us!

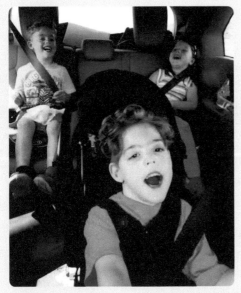

Levi, Cam, and Ana in their first modified minivan.

Adaptive beds and sleep systems

a) Adaptive beds

Adaptive beds, also referred to as hospital beds, are beds specially designed to enhance comfort, positioning, safety, and care. The features of an adaptive bed include adjustable elevation of the head and foot of the bed; adjustable height for the whole bed (manual or electronic); full or half rails and pads; and wheels (which are lockable) to assist bed mobility.

Adaptive beds are used when the individual cannot be positioned well or safely in a typical bed with pillows and wedges. They offer many benefits, including repositioning for comfort and pressure relief, elevating the head to accommodate respiratory or digestive conditions, and elevating the feet to relieve pressure on the heels. Bedrails provide safety, and the adjustable height eases caregiving and accessibility for transfers. A bed that features remote control height adjustment allows the individual more control to assist, for example, with level transfers to and from their wheelchair and to help with care. The adjustable bed height also helps with dressing, bowel and bladder management, and tube feedings.*

There are two types of adaptive bed mattresses:

- Group 1 mattresses and overlays (pad on top of standard mattress) are the least costly of pressure-reducing sleep surfaces and are made from foam, gel, or air.
- Group 2 mattresses and overlays that offer a greater level of pressure reduction include **alternating air mattresses** and **low-air-loss mattresses**.[197]
  - **Alternating air mattresses** are designed with a series of air cells that inflate and deflate in a cyclical pattern. This helps regularly redistribute the weight of the individual, reducing pressure on specific areas of the body, which helps in the prevention of pressure ulcers.
  - **Low-air-loss mattresses** are designed to maintain a constant flow of air through the mattress surface. This airflow helps to manage moisture and temperature, keeping the individual's skin dry and cool, which helps in the prevention and treatment of pressure ulcers.

b) Sleep systems

While focus of postural care is typically on waking hours, nighttime postural care focuses on posture for sleep time.[197] If pillows, wedges, blankets, and other supports do not allow the individual to achieve good posture and comfort throughout the night, a sleep system might be considered. A sleep system is a specialized arrangement of positioning aids designed to optimize comfort and promote proper posture during sleep for individuals with disabilities. Nighttime stretching may also be included. Figures 4.4.4 and 4.4.5 show supine-lying and side-lying sleep systems. A third option, not shown, is a prone-lying sleep system.

---

* There are various other specialty beds that offer features for positioning safety, and comfort. An evaluation with an occupational therapist or your medical provider is recommended if it is determined a standard hospital bed will not meet the needs of the individual. It should be noted that in the US, insurance coverage for these options is often very limited.

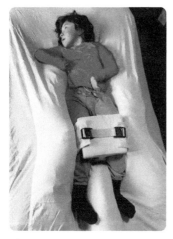

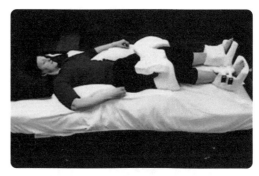

Figure 4.4.4 Supine-lying sleep systems. Right image reproduced with kind permission from Dr. Jennifer Hutson.

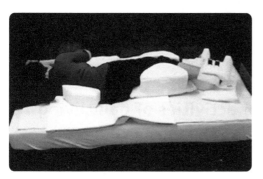

Figure 4.4.5 Side-lying sleep system. Reproduced with kind permission from Dr. Jennifer Hutson.

Levi has had a variety of sleep systems. For a very long time, he had a simple medical bed with metal side rails that had pads attached. As he grew bigger and we recognized that he was not sleeping well, we tried different mattresses. We added a foam mattress and then trialed a sleep system with Velcro supports, but it wasn't right for Levi. Next we trialed the Prius Rhythm Turn Mattress System—an inflated mattress topper that can be programmed either to stay stable or alternate the air through chambers to softly turn the person. This system worked for Levi. We did need many positioning pillows to lift his feet and hold his legs and arms. What we found to be most effective were weighted stuffed animals. He usually has a small zoo of animals stuffed around his body as he sleeps!

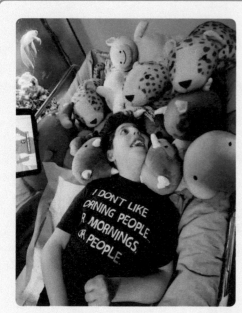

Levi's sleep system.

Adaptive equipment for activities of daily living

Adaptive equipment for activities of daily living (ADLs) includes specialized tools designed to help individuals perform everyday tasks such as taking a shower, eating a meal, and getting dressed. These tools are designed to compensate for limitations in motor control and can help to promote independence and participation. There are many types of adaptive equipment for ADLs; some are described below, including:

a) **Adaptive bathroom equipment**
b) **Eating, drinking, and dressing aids**
c) **Digital accessibility features and tools**

a) Adaptive bathroom equipment

Adaptive bathroom equipment helps to improve accessibility, function, and safety during activities such as bathing and toileting. See Table 4.4.3.

Table 4.4.3 Adaptive bathroom equipment

TYPE	DESCRIPTION	IMAGE
Bathtub chair	This supportive chair is typically made with PVC or metal and mesh. It can be simple or include many supports, such as a head support, lateral support, pelvic positioner, and leg supports. It typically includes back angle adjustment for positioning and accessories such as a bathtub stand to raise the chair height for caregiver access and transfer safety. A bathtub chair is often used when a child outgrows a commercial bathtub support but continues to require specialized positioning in the tub.	
Bathtub lift	This waterproof chair has an electronic remote control to raise it to the level of the bathtub's edge and lower it onto the bathtub floor. It is often made of a combination of plastic, metal, foam, and mesh materials, and can be removed and replaced if the bathtub is a shared space. It can be a good option to increase bathtub transfer safety and caregiver strain. This option can be beneficial for those who benefit from soaking in warm water to reduce spasticity and pain.	
Bathtub transfer system	This system includes a rolling shower/commode chair (i.e., it has wheels or casters) and a track system in which the seat slides into and over the tub. This allows an individual to take a shower sitting in a supportive chair in the bathtub. Often, this is a great choice for someone unsafe to transfer onto a bathtub-based chair but who does not have access to a roll-in shower.	

Cont'd.

TYPE	DESCRIPTION	IMAGE
Commode/ shower chair	This portable chair has a hole in the seat and a container beneath it, designed for individuals who have difficulty accessing a regular toilet. It can be used as a standalone commode or be rolled (it has casters or wheels) to be used as a shower chair in a roll-in shower.	

Bathtub lift reproduced with kind permission from Clarke Healthcare. Bathtub transfer system reproduced with kind permission from Showerbuddy.

> When Levi was a toddler, he had an adaptive toilet seat.* We could hold him on it, and he would use the bathroom. This was a great help, especially when he was constipated, but as he grew older and bigger, it was too difficult to hold him up on the toilet.

b) Eating, drinking, and dressing aids

Eating and drinking aids are specialized tools designed to help with self-feeding. Dressing aids are tools designed to make clothing easier to put on. Clothing and footwear may also be designed to be more accessible. See Table 4.4.4.

---

* An adaptive toilet seat typically fits over an existing toilet seat to provide additional support and comfort.

Table 4.4.4 Eating, drinking, and dressing aids

TYPE	DESCRIPTION	IMAGE
Adaptive utensils	Utensils with modifications that make them easier for an individual to hold and use. For example, they may have modified handles (e.g., larger or more textured) for an easier grip, or they may have altered weight (lighter or heavier) to compensate for muscle weakness or shaky movements.	
Adaptive cups and straws	Cups and straws with modifications to make them easier to hold and drink from. For example, cups may have lids with straws or smaller openings to help control drinking, or straws may have specialized valves to regulate the flow of liquid.	
Adaptive bowls and plates	Bowls and plates with modifications to allow for easier scooping of food. For example, they may have nonslip bases to prevent the bowl or plate from tipping, or they may have high edges to prevent food from spilling.	
Robotic support options	Robotic-based systems that support self-feeding and drinking. They are typically activated by a switch that can be located in a position accessible to the person. This allows the individual to bring food to their mouth at their own pace and to decrease the support needed at mealtimes.	
Zipper pull	A small, usually metallic or plastic attachment that can be put on the slider of a zipper, making it easier to open and close.	
Shoe horn	A curved or flat implement, usually made of plastic, metal, or horn, that can aid getting the foot into a shoe.	
Dressing stick	A short stick, approximately 2 feet (0.6 meters) with a small metal hook on one end and a rubberized hook on the other to assist with pulling up pants, accessing items from the floor, and completing dressing routine.	

Cont'd.

TYPE	DESCRIPTION	IMAGE
Sock aid	A device that comes in various designs that assists in supporting the sock to allow it to be put on a foot more easily and independently. This can often be helpful with long AFO socks that are more challenging for someone with limited dexterity.	
Reacher	A specialized tool designed to assist in reaching and grasping objects that are out of the person's immediate reach. Reachers come in various lengths and triggers for activation. These can support accessing clothing from a closet or floor and sometimes with pulling up pants	
Adaptive clothing and footwear	Specially designed garments and shoes tailored to accommodate the needs of individuals with disabilities. Many companies are now creating clothing and footwear with universal design in mind to be accessible to all. This includes zipper or Velcro closures for shoes, and poncho-style winter coats that are wheelchair friendly and have magnetic and Velcro closures (instead of buttons). These increase accessibility and independence.	

c) Digital accessibility features and tools

Digital accessibility features and tools are continually evolving and increasing in availability. They enable individuals to better access and use technology such as computers, phones, or tablets. To learn what's available, seeking support from an occupational or recreational therapist is recommended. Examples include:

- Devices with built-in accessibility features, such as a tablet with the option to display volume controls as on-screen buttons instead of pressing small, physical buttons, or web browsers with accessibility features, such as keyboard shortcuts instead of operating a mouse
- Adaptive technology tools such as computer keyboards with larger keys for easier use or a screen reader that provides audio output of text displayed on a screen for individuals who have visual impairments
- Options for voice to text to allow access to written communication if hand function does not allow this
- Gaming systems with options such as adaptive game controllers, switch access to use other body parts, voice controls, and eye gaze features to allow players of various abilities to engage in this leisure activity

Some communities have rehabilitation technology specialists or device lending and/or demonstration centers. Check with your community to discover what might be available to trial or purchase.

Augmentative and alternative communication

Augmentative and alternative communication (AAC) describes communication methods that can supplement or compensate for an individual's problems with expressive communication.[199] As we saw in section 2.1, individuals with spastic quadriplegia often face challenges with producing speech. AAC provides a solution to these challenges, allowing individuals to communicate with others. AAC can either be unaided or aided communication.[199] Unaided communication is performed without the use of any tools or technology, such as using gestures, facial expressions, or signs to communicate. Aided communication requires the use of a tool or technology.

Examples of tools and technologies used for aided communication include:

- **Pen and paper:** writing or printing on paper
- **Photographs:** communicating needs through photographs
- **Picture or symbol cards:** communicating using alphabet boards
- **Text-to-speech software:** typing on a device, such as a phone or computer, and using software to generate a computer's voice relaying that text to listeners
- **Eye gaze system:** moving a cursor on a screen using eye movements to select messages or symbols to communicate needs; generally beneficial for individuals with very limited motor movement
- **Tablet or smartphone apps:** using apps with symbol and photograph libraries or text-to-speech software
- **Speech generating device (SGD):** using specialized communication equipment that generates speech from a variety of possible inputs; for example, a person typing on a keyboard, selecting words or phrases from a touch screen, or using switch access; can also incorporate an eye gaze system

Devices used for AAC, such as tablets, smartphones, or SGDs, can be mounted onto mobility devices like wheelchairs or onto rolling mounts for portable use (a frame with wheels that serves as a stand for the device); see Figure 4.4.6. They can also be mounted on tables.

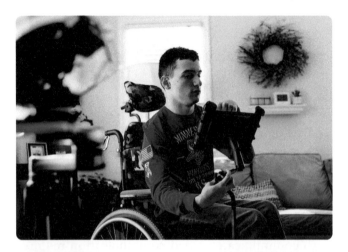

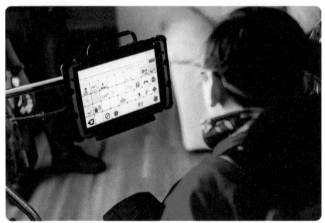

Figure 4.4.6 AAC device on a rolling mount.

Levi uses both a Tobii eye gaze device and manual buttons for AAC. He gets very frustrated with the effort required for AAC speech devices but is gaining some skill in using them. He began using an eye gaze system in elementary school and has continued to practice as he has grown. While the eye gaze seems to be the AAC device best suited for him due to his lack of purposeful motor control for buttons, his vision impairment makes using it very difficult. Levi prefers to use various cries and nonverbal body signals to manipulate those around him to do what he wants! At home we understand what most of his cries mean, and we jump to help him whenever he makes a peep.

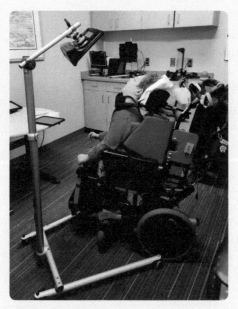

Levi in his wheelchair with his Tobii eye gaze device.

Environmental control devices

Environmental control devices allow an individual to control their environment independently, such as lighting or temperature settings in the home. An example is technology such as Amazon's Alexa Smart Home, which uses voice commands to lock the front door, turn on the TV, or adjust the temperature setting. Many of these technologies can be operated through adaptive control mechanisms such as pointers or eye gaze tracking in addition to voice commands.

Orthoses

Orthoses are designed to hold specific body parts in position in order to modify their structure and/or function. The term "orthosis" comes from the Greek word "ortho," which means "to straighten or align." Orthotics is the branch of medicine concerned with the design, manufacture, and management of orthoses. The orthotist is the professional in this specialty. The word "orthotic" is sometimes used to mean the device; "orthosis" is the more correct term, but given how alike the two terms are, their interchangeability is understandable. The terms "brace" and "splint" are also sometimes used. Orthoses work best when a child has no contractures or bone torsions, though many children with spastic quadriplegia may have both.

Different orthoses have different functions. The goals of treatment with orthoses may include some of the following:[197]

- Maintain or improve ROM at a joint through a prolonged stretch
- Provide stability or support to a joint
- Improve function
- Provide protection
- Accommodate or minimize a joint alignment problem
- Prepare for surgery
- Facilitate positioning after surgery

Choosing an orthosis involves collaboration of many members of the team—often including the orthotist, therapist, physician, and family. Collaborative goal-setting is important[200] as there is frequently a trade-off with orthoses. For example, using a spinal orthosis to help stabilize a person during sitting activities may weaken their independent trunk strength when not wearing it. This is an example of how there may be competing goals in the treatment plan, with no perfect solution: on one hand, we may want to offer support for the trunk during some activities, and on the other hand, we want to see the person work on strengthening their trunk muscles. A balance between the goals and their interventions must be identified, with the understanding that a perfect orthosis for all goals rarely exists.

Orthoses can be custom-made (molded to a specific individual's body) or prefabricated (fit based on size and already made). Different orthoses may be prescribed over the years as the child or adolescent grows and their goals and their body structure and function changes. A custom device such as an ankle-foot orthosis (AFO) requires that a mold first be taken; then the individual returns in a couple of weeks to be fitted with the new orthosis. Adjustments are made to confirm that it fits comfortably and functions well. Adherence to the prescribed wear time is critical to ensure that the individual receives the full benefit of the device. After the initial fitting, further adjustments may be needed if the individual is experiencing:

- Discomfort
- Redness of the skin
- Skin breakdown
- A growth spurt
- A change in functionality
- A change in ROM

Children will likely outgrow their devices before they wear them out and may require new devices every year or so until they stop growing.

This section addresses the types of orthoses individuals with spastic quadriplegia may use:

a) **Lower extremity orthoses**
b) **Upper extremity orthoses**
c) **Body support orthoses**

a) Lower extremity orthoses

Lower extremity orthoses are used for the feet, ankles, knees, and hips. They are intended to maintain ROM at the joint but also provide support and positioning during standing, therapeutic walking, or transfers that require bearing weight on the lower extremities. The following are types of lower extremity orthoses that may be used in spastic quadriplegia and are explained in Table 4.4.5:

- Ankle-foot orthosis (AFO)
- Knee immobilizer (KI)
- Knee orthosis (KO)
- Hip abduction pillow

Shoes that fit well must be worn with orthoses intended for standing or therapeutic walking. If the shoes do not fit well, the orthoses may not function correctly and may not be comfortable. In most cases, a slightly larger shoe is needed. Certain stores including some online allow purchase of two different sized shoes. Athletic shoes that can be zipped, laced, or fastened snugly can be a good option. Some manufacturers of athletic shoes now offer models that are specifically designed to be easy to get on and off with orthoses, such as some BILLY shoes or the Nike FlyEase.

Table 4.4.5 Common lower extremity orthoses used to treat spastic quadriplegia

ORTHOSIS TYPE	SUBTYPE	DESCRIPTION
Ankle-foot orthosis (AFO) An AFO extends above the ankle joint and stops before the knee. It protects the foot, manages foot malalignments, prevents the toes from dragging during gait, provides support and stability to the ankle and/or knee during standing and walking, and prevents the progression of ankle muscle contractures.	Articulated AFO 	An articulated AFO has a hinge at the ankle joint to allow free dorsiflexion (moving the foot up). It often has a plastic posterior "stop" that blocks plantar flexion, preventing the user from moving the foot down or dragging their toes. Articulated AFOs are also worn by those who would benefit from the added ROM while still preventing their toes from dragging.
	Solid AFO (SAFO) 	A SAFO is the most supportive type of AFO. It is typically made of a rigid, durable plastic and provides maximum stability for the ankle and knee. This AFO does not allow ankle movement, which can make some functional movements difficult to perform while wearing it (e.g., getting up from the floor). It is most often recommended for individuals with severe tone, significant weakness, rigid deformities, and/or those who are nonambulatory.
	Nighttime AFO or stretching splint 	A prefabricated nighttime AFO typically has a plastic shell, soft inner liner, and adjustable straps. It is worn just at night and is designed to help stretch the calf muscles, maintain ankle ROM, and prevent the progression of ankle muscle contractures.

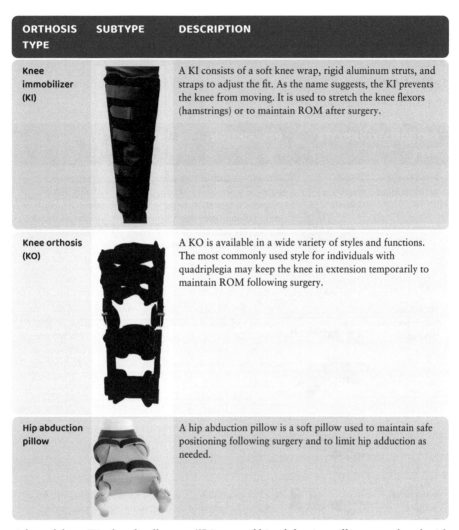

ORTHOSIS TYPE	SUBTYPE	DESCRIPTION
Knee immobilizer (KI)		A KI consists of a soft knee wrap, rigid aluminum struts, and straps to adjust the fit. As the name suggests, the KI prevents the knee from moving. It is used to stretch the knee flexors (hamstrings) or to maintain ROM after surgery.
Knee orthosis (KO)		A KO is available in a wide variety of styles and functions. The most commonly used style for individuals with quadriplegia may keep the knee in extension temporarily to maintain ROM following surgery.
Hip abduction pillow		A hip abduction pillow is a soft pillow used to maintain safe positioning following surgery and to limit hip adduction as needed.

Adapted from Ward and colleagues.[197] Image of hip abduction pillow reproduced with kind permission from Enovis.

b) Upper extremity orthoses

Upper extremity orthoses are used for the fingers, hands, wrists, elbows, and shoulders. They are intended to maintain ROM of the joint, to provide support, and/or to maximize positioning and function. The following are types of upper extremity orthoses that may be used in spastic quadriplegia and are explained in Table 4.4.6:

- Hand finger orthosis (HFO)
- Wrist hand finger orthosis (WHFO)

- Wrist hand orthosis (WHO)
- Elbow orthosis (EO)

Table 4.4.6 Common upper extremity orthoses for individuals with spastic quadriplegia.

ORTHOSIS TYPE	SUBTYPE	DESCRIPTION
Hand finger orthosis (HFO)	Thumb abduction orthosis	A thumb abduction orthosis covers the hand and thumb. It can be made from rigid thermoplastic* or softer, flexible neoprene material. It supports the thumb joint in a functional grasp position, preventing hypermobility, and can be useful during play activities. It also prevents the thumb from coming into the palm during fisting.
Wrist hand finger orthosis (WHFO)	Static	A static WHFO holds the wrist, hand, and fingers in one position and does not allow movement. The rigidity of the material can vary, and it may be worn at night or at rest due to its impact on the user's functionality. It is typically used to counteract or prevent painful wrist and/or finger contractures.
	Dynamic	A dynamic WHFO helps to position the wrist, hand, and fingers while allowing movement to improve overall function.
Wrist hand orthosis (WHO)		A WHO covers only the wrist and hand (not the fingers). It can be made of a variety of materials including neoprene, nylon, thermoplastic,* or metal. A WHO helps to maintain wrist positioning while allowing finger flexion and thumb opposition (touching the tip of the thumb to the tip of the fingers).
Elbow orthosis (EO)		An EO (or elbow immobilizer) is worn around the elbow joint. There are a variety of options, from static EOs that maintain one position to counteract flexion contractures and protect the joint to dynamic EOs that allow movement and can improve ROM. The image is of a static EO.

* Thermoplastic material becomes more pliable when heated and is therefore useful for making or adjusting orthoses.

Adapted from Ward and colleagues.[197] Dynamic WHFO image reproduced with kind permission from Saebo Inc.

When Levi was young, he had thumb orthoses (Benik splints) and AFOs. As he grew older, he stopped using the thumb splints and would cry when we put on his AFOs. Eventually, he would wear the AFOs only in the stander, and by middle school he would not tolerate them at all. For Levi, the splints and AFOs did not prevent deformity or contracture; they simply caused him pain. As he is nonambulatory, the benefits did not outweigh his hatred of them. By age 10, he was done with orthoses. After he had hip and spinal surgeries, Levi was given a hip abduction pillow and knee immobilizers to use while he was healing. My suggestion if you have a child in diapers using a hip abduction pillow is to always put a barrier between the diaper and the pillow because those pillows are nearly impossible to launder!

c) Body support orthoses

Individuals with spastic quadriplegia often require additional support for their head and trunk (neck and/or core muscles) to engage in sitting and mobility activities.

i) Neck support orthoses
Figure 4.4.7 shows a simple neck collar that provides extra neck support to help keep the head upright.

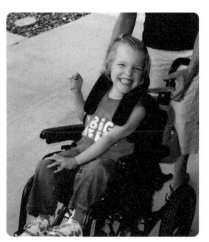 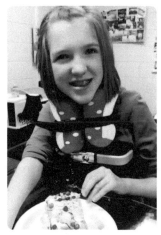

Figure 4.4.7 Neck support orthoses. (In the image on the right, the neck collar is covered with knee-high socks.)

ii) Trunk support orthoses

Trunk supports can range from a basic abdominal binder to a trunk orthosis with metal stays or thermoplastic components. Depending on the specific needs, the trunk support can be customized to support certain muscle groups to enable greater independence with sitting and body control for activity engagement and strengthening. An example is a Benik neoprene body suit (see Figure 4.4.8).

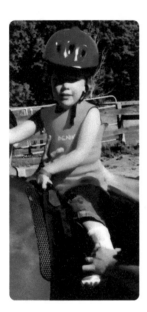 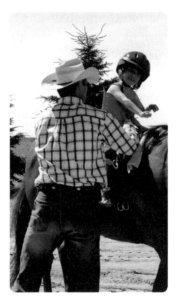

Figure 4.4.8 Trunk support orthosis.

Orthoses for scoliosis management are further addressed in Appendix 4 (online).

Levi has very little head and trunk control, so he has always needed support. Various wheelchair attachments have been useful to hold his head up, though as you can tell in most of his pictures, we are still searching for the perfect solution. A simple airplane pillow can be a great support, and it's an inexpensive and easy-to-find help!

Adaptive recreational equipment

A variety of adaptive recreational equipment is available to make participation in various recreational or leisure pursuits possible or just even easier. An appointment with a recreational therapist, physical therapist, or occupational therapist is useful if people need guidance. Examples of such equipment follow here:

a) Cycles
b) Adaptive workout equipment
c) Hiking aids
d) Other outdoor and adventure sports equipment
e) Technology options
f) Adaptive art and crafts equipment
g) Reading options
h) Adaptive equipment for games

a) Cycles

Adaptive cycles come in many configurations, but for the individual with quadriplegia, an adaptive tricycle allows for more stability to accommodate for balance challenges. Consideration of the transfer height to the cycle seat and the center of gravity while riding may be factors in choosing an upright style versus a recumbent* style. Other factors affecting choice include the age, size, and abilities of the cyclist. Features such as foot plates (also known as shoe holders) with straps, trunk positioning options (such as lateral pads, lap belt, and chest harness), or headrests allow for optimal safety and function. Additionally, a caregiver steering column allows for safety and control by a caregiver assisting with the steering and braking. Integration into family activities is important, so for longer rides or situations where pedaling is less important than inclusion, other cycle styles are available for the rider to simply enjoy the ride. These cycles or trailers may attach to a standard adult cycle, or there are tandem options where the wheelchair can be toted along too. See Figures 4.4.9 and 4.4.10.

---

* Where the cyclist is seated in a reclined or lying-back position.

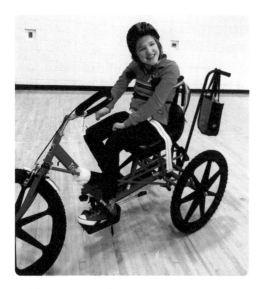

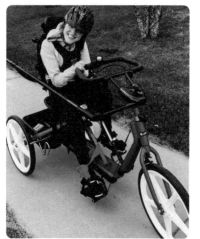

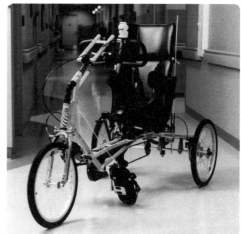

Figure 4.4.9 Foot-powered adaptive tricycles.

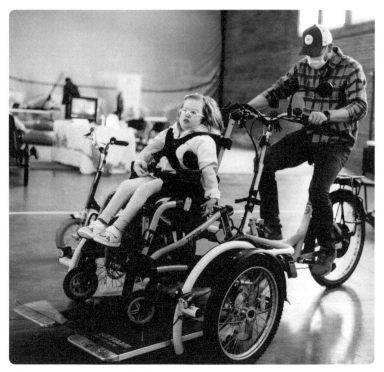

Figure 4.4.10 A non-pedaling rider tandem adaptive cycle.

b) Adaptive workout equipment

Weight-lifting exercises may be done safely with adaptive equipment such as a wrist cuff grip to hold a free weight. They can also be done with a regular wrist weight that goes around the wrist or by using resistance bands. See Figure 4.4.11.

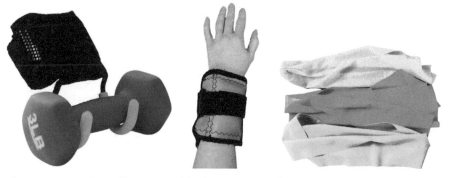

Figure 4.4.11 Wrist cuff grip to hold a free weight (left), wrist weight (middle), and resistance bands (right).

c) Hiking aids

There are some wearable riding options with higher weight capacities to allow a larger child or a smaller adult to ride on a caregiver's back to enjoy the outdoors.

Another option is a pull-behind chariot (a seat on wheels, attached to poles). This is also known as a tandem hiker. See Figure 4.4.12.

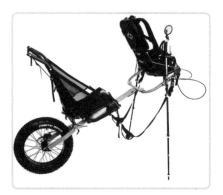 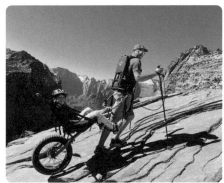

Figure 4.4.12 A pull-behind chariot. Reproduced with kind permission from Huckleberry Hiking.

A track chair is an all-terrain wheelchair that can safely navigate outdoor spaces. Some large parks and recreational facilities have these chairs available to borrow while at the park or at the beach, for example. See Figure 4.4.13.

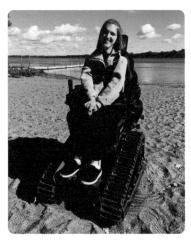 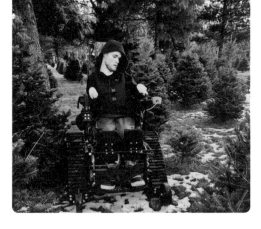

Figure 4.4.13 Track chairs.

d) Other outdoor and adventure sports equipment

Adaptive equipment is available for many other outdoor and adventure sports, including:

- Swimming aids (e.g., an adaptive life jacket with extra head support for floating and/or swimming)
- Jogging strollers
- Frame running (also known as race running), where individuals compete with running frames on an athletics track
- Snow skiing (e.g., outriggers)
- Waterskiing (e.g., arm sling handles, shoulder wraps, sit skis)
- Golf (e.g., adaptive club grips and golf carts)
- Kayaking (e.g., angled oars, outriggers, trolling motors)
- Surfing (e.g., specialized systems)
- Horseback riding (e.g., high back saddles for balance)
- Adaptive baseball (e.g., use of a wrist band to hold the bat)

These can have various levels of assistance and support. See Figures 4.4.14 to 4.4.18.

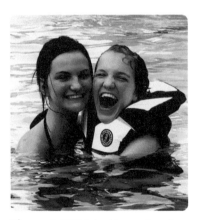
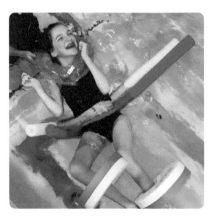

Figure 4.4.14 Adaptive swimming.

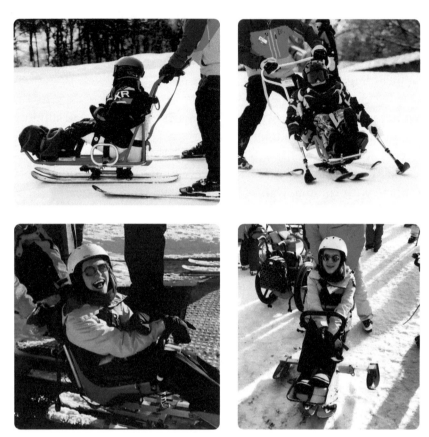

Figure 4.4.15 Adaptive snow skiing.

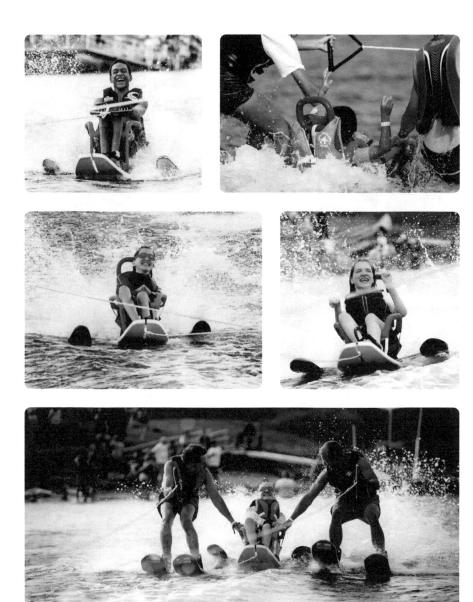

Figure 4.4.16 Adaptive waterskiing.

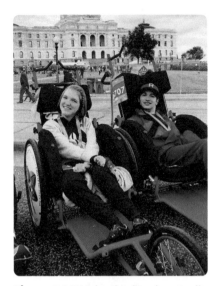
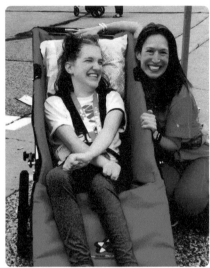

Figure 4.4.17 Adaptive jogging strollers.

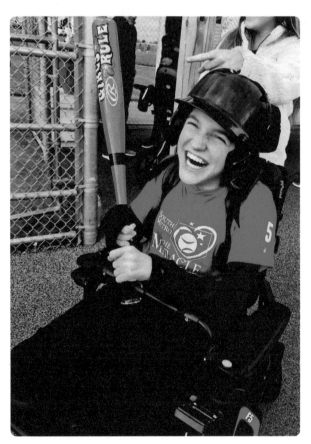

Figure 4.4.18 Adaptive baseball.

e) Technology options

An adaptive joystick and adaptive color-coded keyboard with large keys and letters help with computer use. Other options such as touch screen, eye gaze, voice control, and switch use can help with navigating digital devices, such as computers, tablets, or video games. See Figure 4.4.19.

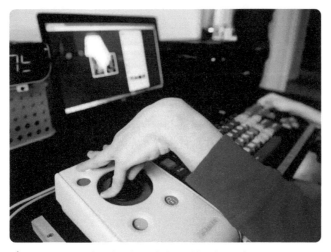

Figure 4.4.19 Adaptive joystick and keyboard.

f) Adaptive art and crafts equipment

Adaptive art and crafts equipment may include:

- Single-extremity scissors with a stability base
- Single-extremity scissors
- Easy-grip scissors
- Universal cuff (can be used for many purposes; here to hold a writing utensil)
- Foam grip aid to assist weak grip
- Paintbrush holder that may prevent fatigue

See Figures 4.4.20 and 4.4.21.

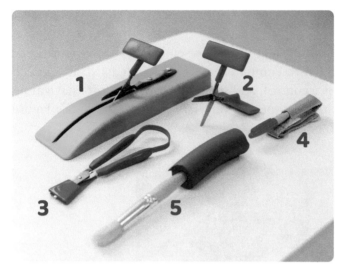

Figure 4.4.20 1) Single-extremity scissors with stability base **2)** Single-extremity scissors **3)** Easy-grip scissors **4)** Universal cuff **5)** Foam grip aid.

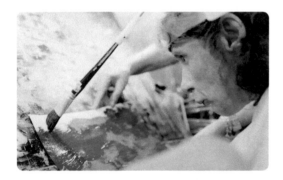

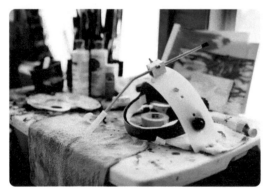

Figure 4.4.21 Paintbrush holder.

g) Reading options

A table-top book stand allows for page turning (see Figure 4.4.22). Alternatively, audiobook options may enhance opportunities to enjoy literature.

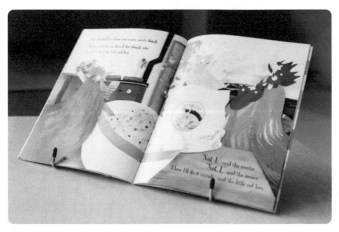

Figure 4.4.22 Table-top book stand.

h) Adaptive equipment for games

Adaptive equipment for playing games may include the following:

- Card shuffler
- Playing card holder
- Adaptive switch for use with a regular bubble-maker
- Dice popper

See Figures 4.4.23 to 4.4.26.

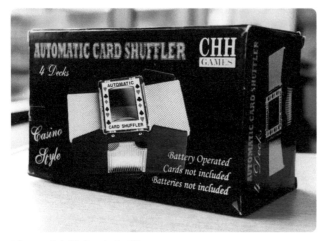

Figure 4.4.23 Card shuffler.

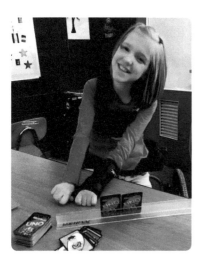

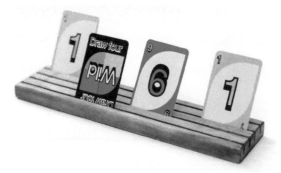

Figure 4.4.24 Playing card holders.

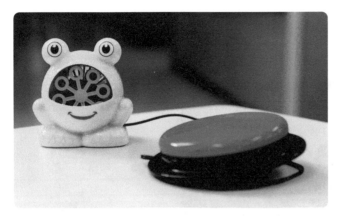

Figure 4.4.25 Adaptive switch for use with a regular bubble-maker.

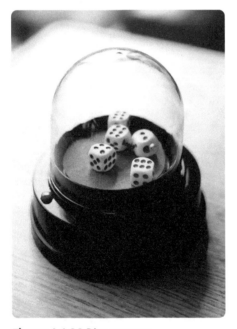

Figure 4.4.26 Dice popper.

The following are photographs of Levi enjoying many recreational activities with his family.

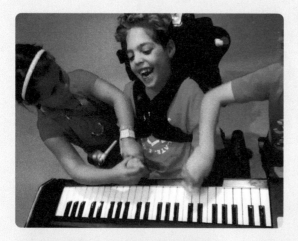
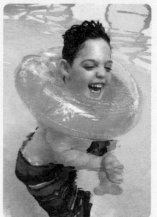
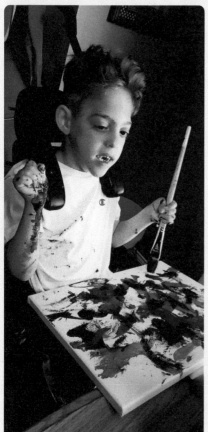
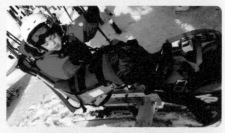
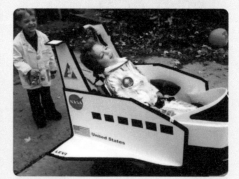
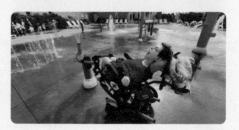

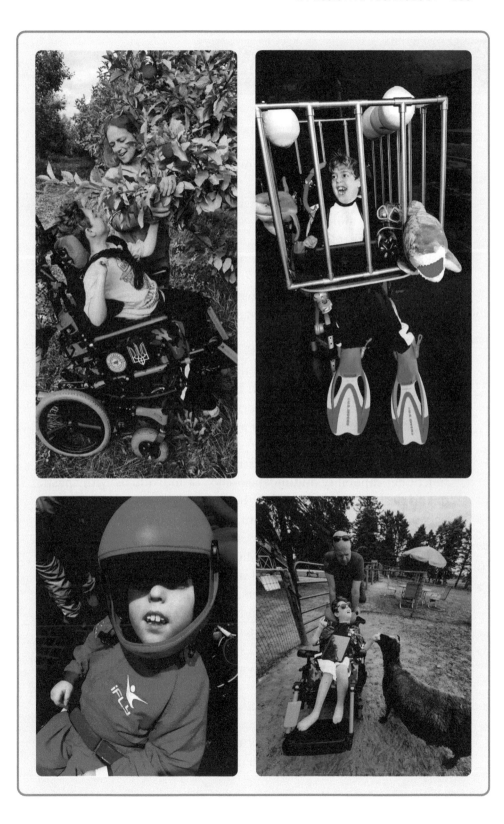

Key points Chapter 4

- Physical therapy, occupational therapy, and/or speech and language pathology (or therapy) are important tools in promoting development and maximizing function for the individual with spastic quadriplegia.
- Physical therapists help the individual to maximize their movement and functional ability.
- Occupational therapists help the individual to complete meaningful tasks and help modify activities or the environment to enable successful task completion.
- Speech and language pathologists/therapists support those with speech, language, and communication needs as well as feeding and swallowing difficulties.
- "It takes a village to raise a child" emphasizes the idea that raising a child, particularly a child with a disability, is not a task that should be shouldered alone by parents. Enlisting the support of others is important. Practicing what is learned in therapy, postural management, and exercise and physical activity are important elements of the home program.
- There is a wide variety of assistive technology that can help the functional capability and independence of individuals with spastic quadriplegia. Therapists and orthotists, together with other members of the multidisciplinary team, work with the individual in this area. Assistive technology includes:
  - Seating, standing, and mobility aids to help improve function during sitting, standing, and movement; these include floor sitters, adaptive chairs, standers, gait trainers, adaptive strollers, wheelchairs, transfer aids, and vehicle transportation
  - Adaptive beds and sleep systems to enhance comfort, positioning, safety, and care
  - Adaptive equipment for activities of daily living (ADLs) to help with everyday tasks, such as adaptive bathroom equipment; eating, drinking, and dressing aids; and digital accessibility features and tools
  - Augmentative and alternative communication (AAC) to supplement or compensate for problems with expressive communication

- ○ Environmental control devices to allow for independent control of the environment
- ○ Orthoses to hold specific body parts in position in order to modify their structure and/or function, including lower and upper extremity and spinal orthoses
- ○ Adaptive recreational equipment to make participation in a wide range of hobbies and sports possible or just even easier

Chapter 5

Managing musculoskeletal health— orthopedic care

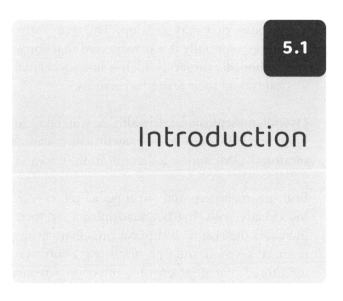

Introduction

Coming together is a beginning;
keeping together is progress;
working together is success.
Edward Everett Hale

This chapter addresses level 3 considerations—managing musculoskeletal health in individuals with spastic quadriplegia. The overall goal of managing musculoskeletal health (i.e., orthopedic care) is to prevent and treat musculoskeletal problems that may interfere with function, ease of daily cares,* and comfort now or in the future to allow the individual to participate as fully as possible in life.

The following topics are addressed in detail in the sections below:

- **Tone reduction,** which may be achieved with interventions ranging from a comprehensive home program to neurosurgery. (Neurosurgery is surgery carried out on the nervous system.)

---

* Daily activities such as dressing, feeding, toileting, and cutting nails, completed by the individual themselves, or supported by a caregiver.

- **Musculoskeletal surveillance,** which involves regular monitoring and assessment of musculoskeletal development and function to watch for problems such as contractures, hip displacement, and scoliosis that may develop. The term "surveillance" means monitoring, especially if it is suspected that something may happen.
- **Orthopedic surgery,** which is surgery carried out on muscles, bones, joints, and their related structures.

Overall musculoskeletal health is watched closely throughout childhood and adolescence, as growth spurts can cause a loss of range of motion (ROM) and/or a deterioration in tone control.

Both neurosurgery and orthopedic surgery are big undertakings for individuals with spastic quadriplegia as their general health status increases the risk of complications. Preoperative general health status must be assessed and optimized (e.g., nutrition and respiratory status monitored, potential sites for infection screened, presence of anemia* checked, constipation addressed). The focus must be on excellent postoperative care.[137] Possible complications include (but are not limited to) increased risks of:

- Anesthesia-related complications due to underlying respiratory problems
- Challenges with postoperative pain management due to heightened sensitivity and limited communication abilities
- Pressure ulcers due to malpositioning, cast pressure, or nutritional deficiencies
- Development or worsening of existing contractures due to prolonged immobilization during the recovery period
- Infection, particularly in those with underlying respiratory or nutritional problems
- Development or worsening of existing feeding, swallowing, nutrition, and digestive problems
- Development or worsening of existing anxiety issues

USEFUL WEB RESOURCES

---

* A condition characterized by a deficiency of red blood cells or hemoglobin in the blood.

Tone reduction

The good physician treats the disease; the great
physician treats the patient who has the disease.
Sir William Osler

Abnormal muscle tone is addressed in section 2.5. To recap: Muscle tone is the resting tension in a muscle. A range of "normal" muscle tone exists. Tone is considered "abnormal" when it falls outside the range of normal or typical. It can be too low (hypotonia) or too high (hypertonia). Abnormal muscle tone occurs in all types of CP. In children with spastic quadriplegia, tone is typically too high in the legs and arms, but it can be low in the trunk.

Recall that data from the Australian CP register shows that 48 percent of individuals with spastic quadriplegia have co-occurring dyskinesia, while 3 percent have co-occurring hypotonia.[42] It is believed that the true prevalence of co-occurring motor types is higher.[4] A more recent study found that 50 percent of children and young people with CP (all types) had spasticity and dystonia. The presence of dystonia with spasticity has been underrecognized.[48] This is important because the management of spasticity and dystonia is different.

Overall goals for tone reduction include:

- Reducing pain
- Improving care, comfort, and positioning
- Improving overall relaxation and sleep quality
- Improving function
- Improving tolerance for wearing orthoses
- Reducing stiffness and increasing the overall ROM of joints
- Reducing the contribution of tone to musculoskeletal problems

Treatment of high tone in children and adolescents with spastic quadriplegia can be accomplished with a variety of interventions. Before determining the treatment plan, goals with the input of the individual (where possible), their family, and members of the multidisciplinary team should be established. The most appropriate tone-reducing treatment for the individual will be chosen.

Many medical centers have special team evaluations of hypertonia because of its complexity and significance in CP. At Gillette Children's, for example, several professionals work together at a spasticity evaluation or movement disorders clinic. The medical professionals on the multidisciplinary team include specialists in physical medicine and rehabilitation (PM&R), orthopedics, neurology, neurosurgery, and rehabilitation therapies. They see the child together, not individually, and come to a consensus opinion on the best treatment plan. Spasticity clinics at other facilities may include other specialties; for example, developmental pediatrics. Rehabilitation after tone reduction is based on the goals of the treatment. Treatment of high tone has traditionally followed a pyramid approach, beginning with the least invasive treatment, moving up the pyramid if adequate tone reduction is not achieved.

- The base of the pyramid is the **daily home stretching program, casting, and/or orthotics** (e.g., AFOs, knee immobilizers, and abduction pillows).
- The next tier is **oral* or enteral[†] medications,** including baclofen, diazepam, and others.

---

* Taken by mouth

† Administered via the feeding tube that delivers nutrition directly into the stomach or small intestine.

- Next is **injectable medications,** including botulinum neurotoxin A (BoNT-A) and phenol.
- The top tier of the pyramid is **neurosurgery,** including intrathecal baclofen, rhizotomy, and deep brain stimulation.

However, rather than thinking of this process as tiers of a pyramid, it is better to think of it as a Venn diagram where many modalities are used together at different times. (See Figure 5.2.1). It is not at all uncommon to use oral or enteral medications in combination with injectable medications, while still doing a stretching program and orthoses. Finally, even after undergoing surgical interventions, medications may be needed. A stretching program and orthoses are typically recommended at all ages.

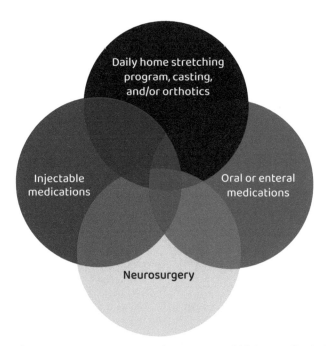

Figure 5.2.1 Venn diagram of treatment of high tone for individuals with spastic quadriplegia.

Any neurosurgery for an individual with spastic quadriplegia should be embarked upon after an appropriate cost-benefit analysis; the potential risks and pain from the procedure itself and its recovery should be weighed against any potential benefit that the individual may receive from that intervention.

Table 5.2.1 explains tone reduction treatments commonly used in spastic quadriplegia.

Table 5.2.1 Tone reduction treatments

TYPE	TREATMENT	GENERALIZED OR FOCAL Generalized = treatment affects a large region of the body. Focal = treatment has an effect on a local area (e.g., a single muscle)	DURATION OF EFFECT	TONE TYPE	HOSPITAL STAY REQUIRED
Oral or enteral medications	Various (see below)	Generalized	Temporary	Spasticity Dystonia	No
Injectable medications	Botulinum neurotoxin A (BoNT-A) injection	Focal: injected into muscles	Temporary	Spasticity*	No
	Phenol injection	Focal: injected around nerves that control spastic muscles	Temporary	Spasticity	No
Neuro-surgery	Intrathecal baclofen (ITB)	Generalized	Temporary	Spasticity Dystonia Choreo-athetosis	Yes
	Ventral dorsal rhizotomy (VDR)	Generalized (lower limbs only)	Permanent	Spasticity Dystonia	Yes
	Deep brain stimulation (DBS)	Focal or generalized	Temporary	Spasticity Dystonia Choreo-athetosis	Yes

* Botulinum neurotoxin A (BoNT-A) may sometimes be used to treat pain caused by dystonia in some individuals with spastic quadriplegia.

The American Academy for Cerebral Palsy and Developmental Medicine (AACPDM) has published a care pathway, "Cerebral Palsy and Dystonia," and a link to it is included in **Useful web resources.**

Oral or enteral medications

There are several oral or enteral medications that physicians may prescribe to reduce spasticity and dystonia, including:

- Baclofen (spasticity and dystonia)
- Diazepam (spasticity)
- Dantrolene sodium (spasticity)
- Tizanidine (spasticity)
- Carbidopa and levodopa (dystonia)
- Trihexyphenidyl (dystonia)
- Tetrabenazine (dystonia)

These medications act at different sites within the body, with different effects on the muscles, brain, or spinal cord.[201] They may have different brand names in different countries. The challenge of treatment with oral or enteral medications is managing their side effects, and some individuals respond better to the medications than others. They are sometimes used in combination or in conjunction with focal spasticity reduction measures such as BoNT-A and phenol. They can also sometimes be used intermittently to reduce muscle spasms; for example, after orthopedic surgery.

Injectable medications

a) Botulinum neurotoxin A injection

Botulinum neurotoxin A (BoNT-A), as a medication, is injected directly into the muscle and acts by blocking the release of a chemical called acetylcholine at the neuromuscular junction (where the nerve meets the muscle). Botulinum neurotoxin[*] is produced by the bacteria that causes botulism, a lethal form of food poisoning. However, as a medication,

---

[*] A poison that acts on the nervous system.

the purified toxin is delivered at a much smaller dose. There are seven different types of botulinum neurotoxin, from A to G. Type A is the main form used to reduce spasticity.[202]

The effects of BoNT-A become apparent approximately three to seven days after injection and last for approximately three to six months.[203] Different institutions may have different protocols for use of BoNT-A (e.g., regarding dosage and frequency of injection).[204] The effects of BoNT-A diminish with time. The original nerves regain their ability to release acetylcholine, but conflicting evidence exists on its long-term effect on the muscle itself.[202,203]

Several muscles may be treated in one session, although there is a limit to the total body dose of BoNT-A that can be safely given at one time.[202] Depending on the the age of the individual and the number of muscles being injected, anesthesia may be required. Typically, no overnight hospital stay is necessary.

As with any injection, there may be some pain associated with the needle puncturing the skin and the delivery of the medicine. Different centers use different methods to manage pain; these may include distraction techniques (e.g., watching a video), topical or oral medication, nitrous oxide (laughing gas), or general anesthesia. Some children may experience stress and anxiety from repeated episodes of injection. One limiting factor of this treatment is that children may experience diminishing effects with repeat injections, or it may stop being effective entirely.[202]

While there is strong evidence supporting BoNT-A treatment,[14,205,206] concerns are being raised. BoNT-A is regarded as a temporary treatment for reducing spasticity, but important questions have been asked about its long-term effects, including muscle weakness, muscle atrophy (wastage), changes in the muscle structure, and atrophy of the underlying bone.[3,203,207–213] Some studies suggest there may be permanent changes. For example, Multani and colleagues reported that human volunteers and experimental animals show muscle atrophy after BoNT-A for at least 12 months.[203] They added that "muscle atrophy was accompanied by loss of contractile elements in muscle and replacement with fat and connective tissue," and that it was not currently known if these changes are reversible. They concluded that there is a need to use BoNT-A "more thoughtfully, less frequently and with greatly enhanced monitoring of

the effects on injected muscle for both short-term and long-term benefits and harms."[203]

b) Phenol injection

Phenol is another medication delivered by injection. It was used as a
treatment for spasticity for many decades before the advent of BoNT-A.
Phenol is injected directly around the motor nerve,[*] causing a breakdown of the insulation around the nerve, which prevents the nerve from
sending messages to the muscle. (Note that phenol is injected around
the nerve, whereas BoNT-A is injected into the muscle.) Treatment with
phenol is normally done under general anesthesia to minimize both
discomfort for the patient and movement during the injection process.
Usually, two to four muscle groups are treated in a single session.

Side effects of phenol may include paresthesia (a pins-and-needles or
burning sensation that happens if sensory nerves are affected instead
of just the motor nerves) and weakness. The paresthesia may last a
few weeks and is treated with gabapentin. The weakness usually
resolves within two to four weeks. Again, no overnight hospital stay is
typically necessary.

The effects of phenol generally last 3 to 12 months. Repeated injections
can lead to a cumulative effect, meaning the effects may last longer than
one year,[202] but this is not common.

The use of phenol differs around the world. It has become less popular
for a number of reasons, including the advent of BoNT-A.[202] Sometimes
it is used in conjunction with BoNT-A because it allows more muscles to be treated without exceeding the dosage recommendations for
either medication.[191] Some centers may use other alcohols in addition
to phenol.

There is only one study supporting phenol use in CP.[14] This is an example
of a situation where there is a lack of research evidence but clinical expertise supports its use.

---

[*] A motor nerve sends signals away from the brain and spinal cord to a muscle. A sensory nerve
sends signals (about temperature, pain, touch, etc.) from all parts of the body to the spinal cord
and brain.

Neurosurgery

Neurosurgery may be considered for individuals with spastic quadri-plegia levels IV and V. The most appropriate neurosurgical procedure for the individual is chosen based on the goals, tone type, and resources available. As mentioned already, neurosurgery is a big undertaking for individuals with spastic quadriplegia as their general health status is often more difficult to maintain and the risk of complication is high.

a) Intrathecal baclofen

Intrathecal baclofen (ITB) is another method for delivering the medica-tion baclofen. The following is an explanation of each term:

- **Intrathecal:** "Intra" means "within," and the "theca" is the sheath enclosing the spinal cord. The intrathecal area is the fluid-filled space surrounding the spinal cord; cerebrospinal fluid flows through this area, bathing and protecting the spinal cord.
- **Baclofen:** The name of the medication.

With ITB, a pump stores and delivers baclofen directly to the cerebro-spinal fluid in the intrathecal space. The pump is filled with baclofen and inserted under the skin and its soft tissue layer, typically in the abdomen. A catheter (a narrow, flexible tube) is connected to the pump and routed under the skin and its soft tissue layer to the patient's back. Surgeons make an incision to thread and position the tip of the cath-eter in the intrathecal space, where it delivers the baclofen directly to the cerebrospinal fluid. The pump is programmed to slowly release baclofen either in a consistent dose or in bursts of medication over the 24-hour period, depending on which method best helps the individual's hypertonia.[214] See Figure 5.2.2.

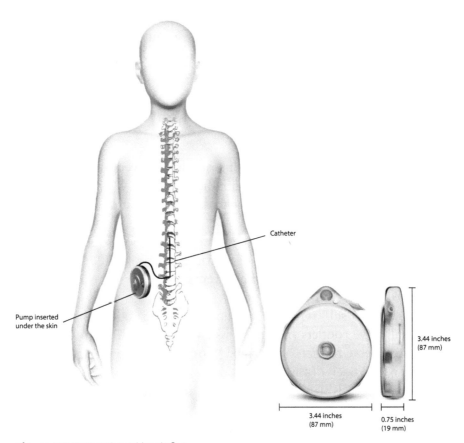

Figure 5.2.2 Intrathecal baclofen.

Delivering baclofen directly into the cerebrospinal fluid is much more effective and requires a much lower dose (about one-thousandth of the oral dose). It can help avoid or minimize side effects that individuals may experience when taking oral baclofen such as dizziness and drowsiness.

Implanting an ITB pump usually requires a hospital stay, typically five to seven days. It is important for the patient to lie flat for up to three days afterwards to allow the surgical site to heal and avoid spinal fluid from leaking. The patient wears an abdominal binder for six to eight weeks afterward to support the pump and prevent swelling.[214] The pump has to be refilled with baclofen about every three to four months, on average, in an outpatient clinic. The pump runs on a battery that has a limited life, requiring the pump to be surgically removed and replaced after about seven years. This can usually be done with an overnight hospital stay.

There is strong evidence supporting the use of intrathecal baclofen for reduced spasticity and/or dystonia in individuals with spastic quadriplegia GMFCS levels IV and V[14] and evidence that it is probably effective for other outcomes.[14]

b) Ventral dorsal rhizotomy

A ventral dorsal rhizotomy is a neurosurgical procedure that reduces spasticity and dystonia by cutting both the dorsal and ventral nerve rootlets in the spinal cord.[215] The following is an explanation of each term:

- **Ventral:** "Ventral" refers to the motor nerve rootlets. Some of the ventral nerve rootlets (i.e., the motor nerve rootlets) are cut. (The motor nerve rootlets are termed "ventral" because they are toward the front of the body.)
- **Dorsal:** "Dorsal" refers to the sensory nerve rootlets. Some of the dorsal nerve rootlets (i.e., the sensory nerve rootlets) are cut. (The sensory nerve rootlets are termed "dorsal" because they are located toward the back of the body).
- **Rhizotomy:** "Rhizo" means "root," and "otomy" means "to cut into."

Putting it all together, "ventral dorsal rhizotomy" means that a percentage of the dorsal and ventral nerve rootlets are cut. Since this is a newer procedure, techniques vary.

A ventral dorsal rhizotomy involves removing the back of the vertebrae (the lamina) to access the spinal cord. During the ventral dorsal rhizotomy, the sensory (dorsal) and motor (ventral) nerve roots are dissected into rootlets.

A ventral dorsal rhizotomy may be considered for individuals who are GMFCS IV or V with significant hypertonia, including spasticity and dystonia that affect their comfort, daily cares, function, and positioning. This procedure can weaken the lower extremities, which can decrease standing ability,[215] so it is important to discuss patient and family goals. Benefits need to be discussed in light of possible negative effects. For example, patients, families, and providers should consider and discuss the degree to which high tone may be useful for helping with transfers or for taking steps, as these may be negatively impacted by the procedure.

Reduction in spasticity and dystonia, improvement in joint ROM in the lower limbs, and functional improvements were found among children with CP with moderate to severe mixed hypertonia (spasticity and dystonia) who underwent a ventral dorsal rhizotomy.[216]

c) Deep brain stimulation

Deep brain stimulation (DBS) is a neurosurgical procedure in which electrodes attached to a flexible wire are placed in the basal ganglia of the brain (important in the control of movement; see Figure 1.2.4). The electrodes are connected to a medical device called a neurostimulator that is implanted under the surface of the skin in the abdomen or chest. (See Figure 5.2.3.) The neurostimulator delivers low-voltage electrical impulses to the brain, which suppress overactive motor nerve cells.

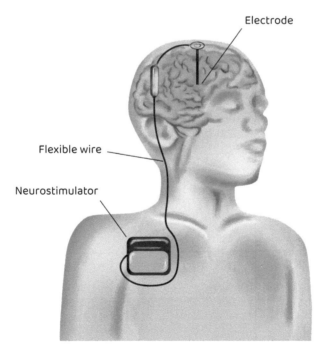

Figure 5.2.3 Deep brain stimulation.

DBS was first developed for use in individuals with Parkinson's disease.* DBS is adjustable (stimulation settings can be changed) and its effect is temporary (the device can be removed without any injury to the brain).[217]

At Gillette Children's, it is common to do the DBS in a two-part surgery. During the first, the electrodes and wires are implanted in both sides of the brain; this typically involves a two-day hospital stay. Then, two weeks later, the neurostimulator is implanted in the abdomen or chest—usually a one- to two-day hospital stay. It can take up to a year to experience the full effects of DBS.[217]

A systematic review found evidence that DBS is possibly effective in reducing dystonia.[218]

Levi has had a lot of tone reduction interventions, including medications and neurosurgery. He does best when we keep up on Botox injections every three months and oral diazepam for the days he has very high tone. We no longer need the phenol injections as his ventral dorsal rhizotomy alleviated the tone in his legs.

---

* A brain disorder that leads to shaking, stiffness, and difficulty with walking, balance, and coordination.

Musculoskeletal surveillance

The greatest medicine of all is teaching people how not to need it.

Hippocrates

Musculoskeletal surveillance is addressed under the following headings:

- Surveillance of lower and upper limb range of motion
- Hip surveillance
- Spine surveillance
- Bone health surveillance

Surveillance of lower and upper limb range of motion

Monitoring of lower and upper limb range of motion (ROM) is an important aspect of musculoskeletal health surveillance. A muscle contracture can limit a joint's ROM. (The terms "muscle contracture" and "tight muscle" are used interchangeably.) Medical professionals routinely measure joint ROM to watch for any deterioration. Typical ROMs for each movement are included in **Useful web resources.**

Hip surveillance

Hip surveillance (monitoring) is very important in the management of children and adolescents with spastic quadriplegia GMFCS levels IV and V because:

- The risk of hip displacement (addressed in section 2.5) is high.
- In the earlier stages, hip displacement is silent (i.e., asymptomatic).
- In earlier stages, reconstructive surgery is more effective than if treated late.
- The consequences of hip displacement are serious.

As was noted in section 2.5, the measure used in X-rays for hip surveillance is called the "migration percentage" (MP), also known as the Reimer's migration index (RMI).

Individuals with spastic quadriplegia spend a large proportion of their day in a seated position, and a dislocated hip (or hips) can be painful while sitting, and over time, any movement of the joint for tasks such as positioning, hygiene, or dressing can also be painful. Health-related quality of life, which is defined as "the way in which a condition (almost always a chronic condition) affects a person's wellbeing,"[8] has been found to be negatively influenced by hip displacement in children with CP GMFCS levels III to V. As well, increasing MP values are correlated with decreasing health-related quality of life.[219]

The goal of hip surveillance is to prevent hip dislocation by early detection and early surgery. For children and adolescents with a diagnosis of CP, hip surveillance should commence immediately at the time of diagnosis. The AACPDM care pathway for individuals with CP GMFCS levels IV and V advises hip surveillance every six months for a minimum of two years until age four and annually after that until skeletal maturity.[220] Each surveillance visit should include clinical examination and X-rays. Once skeletal maturity is reached, annual surveillance should continue if the MP is greater than 30 percent.[220] Similar guidelines exist in other countries. A link to the AACPDM care pathway for individuals with CP is included in **Useful web resources,** and families are encouraged to read it and ensure that hip health is being closely monitored.

The importance of hip surveillance cannot be underestimated. Formal hip surveillance programs exist in some countries (e.g., Sweden and Australia) and have been easier to implement in countries with national health care systems. Ten years after the Swedish surveillance program commenced, the incidence of hip dislocations was reduced from 9.0 percent to 0.4 percent.[221] A 20-year follow-up showed that the number of hip dislocations remained stable.[138] What was learned from the Swedish program is that comprehensive multidisciplinary intervention at the right time and the right dose can prevent hip dislocation.[14]

Levi was followed closely with hip X-rays at least yearly since birth. That frequency increased when there was a noticeable change in his hips coming out of the socket, and he had his first bilateral hip surgery in 2015. He was scheduled for a revision in 2020, but instead had the ventral dorsal rhizotomy, and we have not needed to intervene with his hips in the three years since. He has had his right hip tendon released, which allowed a greater mobility of his right leg, making diapering much easier. This has improved the range of motion of the right hip; however, this area does have a tendency to hold onto moisture and become irritated or yeasty. We have been looking for the right combination of barrier creams and devices such as absorbent pads to prevent skin breakdown in this area. A sanitary napkin seems to do the trick!

Spine surveillance

Like hip surveillance, spine surveillance is also very important because:

- The risk of scoliosis (addressed in section 2.5) is high.
- The consequences of scoliosis are serious.

However, unlike with hip surveillance, no formal guidelines currently exist for spine surveillance. The development of clinical guidelines for scoliosis surveillance has been recommended,[134] so it is likely that they will become available soon.

General recommendations include that X-rays be taken if a new curve in the spine is noticed or if posture has noticeably changed. If a curve is confirmed on X-rays, repeat X-rays should be taken after six months to assess the progression of the curve. Thereafter, continued monitoring of the curve should be performed every 6 to 12 months.

Any curve greater than approximately 20 degrees is ideally followed by a spine specialist who will decide whether to monitor the curve's progress or intervene. Intervention options include a spinal orthosis.* Information on scoliosis management is included in Appendix 4 (online). Spine surgery is typically not considered until the curve reaches a magnitude that is not anticipated to stabilize (approximately 40 degrees) and there is concern that it will continue to progress.

Bone health surveillance

Because of the risk of early osteopenia or osteoporosis, it is recommended that individuals with CP have an annual bone health assessment with appropriate blood testing and imaging. This includes a lifestyle review, nutrition assessment, and, as needed, evaluation for any concerning changes in bone health, such as new fractures or medications that affect bone health. A bone density scan (called a DXA or DEXA†scan) of the spine and hips is not routinely recommended but can be a useful adjunct for surveillance if indicated, depending on the individual's history or risk factors (e.g., if the individual has less dense bones as observed on X-ray or has had fragility fractures). To promote optimum bone health throughout life, good nutrition, ensuring no deficiencies in calcium and vitamin D, and physical activity, especially weight-bearing or impact activities, can help.[222]

The American Academy for Cerebral Palsy and Developmental Medicine (AACPDM) has published a care pathway, "Osteoporosis in Cerebral Palsy," and a link to it is included in **Useful web resources.**

---

* A spinal orthosis (removable brace) that applies corrective forces to the spine to slow or stop scoliosis curve progression.

† Dual-energy X-ray absorptiometry.

Orthopedic surgery

Fractures well cured make us more strong.
Ralph Waldo Emerson

Orthopedic surgery in the management of the musculoskeletal problems in individuals with spastic quadriplegia aims to address current problems and may be useful to prevent future problems. Having a multidisciplinary team and shared goal-setting between the individual with their family and medical professionals is very important, with everyone weighing the benefits and risks of surgical intervention against those of not proceeding with surgery.

As mentioned already, orthopedic surgery is a significant undertaking for individuals with spastic quadriplegia. For them, the risks are higher due to their associated health conditions. The goals for orthopedic surgery include improving function, ease of daily cares, and comfort. If there is not consensus that surgery will achieve these goals, then it is avoided. Otherwise, it becomes somewhat "cosmetic," meaning only the appearance of the limb is being changed, not the function or benefit for the person. Ideally, surgery is contemplated only after less invasive options have first been explored.

Soft tissue surgery can include:

- **Tendon release:** Severing the tendon of a contracted muscle to allow for a greater range of motion of the joint. Once the tendon is severed, the function of the muscle is markedly diminished, which therefore decreases the problematic pull of the muscle.
- **Tendon transfer:** Reattaching the tendon at a different point to change the function of the muscle. For example, a muscle that behaved as a joint flexor, when transferred, could become a joint extensor. The goal is to improve the balance of muscles around a joint.
- **Muscle and/or tendon lengthening:** Lengthening the muscle and/or tendon, though not releasing the tendon entirely, allowing for continued action of that muscle.
- **Muscle recession:** Dividing the sheet of tissue where the muscle ends and the tendon begins. This is most commonly done in the calf, with the sheet of tissue of the gastrocnemius being separated from a similar sheet for the soleus (as they come together at their common Achilles tendon) and only the gastrocnemius tissue (the two-joint muscle) being divided.

It is important to note that with tendon release or muscle and/or tendon lengthening surgery, variable degrees of weakness occur, and with further growth there may be recurrence of the contracture.

It is also worth noting that contractures are surprisingly complicated to alleviate because it frequently requires not just soft tissue (muscle and tendon) surgery, but also bone surgery, making the procedure quite invasive. For this reason, the decision to correct a contracture is not simple, and the benefit to the individual needs to be considered. Will correction of the contracture allow for better function? Will it make daily cares easier? Will it allow for better positioning? If not, it may be appropriate to accept the contracture and instead, for example, use positioning support.

At some centers and in some cases, tendon release and muscle and/or tendon lengthening to relieve contractures is done percutaneously (i.e., a minimal incision through the skin), which is an easier surgery for child or adolescent with spastic quadriplegia. Some centers use percutaneous surgery minimally or not at all due to concerns with the ability to avoid injury to surrounding structures and to control the extent of the surgery.

If the team comes to the consensus that the individual is likely to derive sufficient benefit from surgery, then the collective decision is made to proceed. An example would be in the case of severe knee flexion contractures that limit ability to participate in stand-pivot transfers; in such a case, proceeding with a more extensive surgery may be the correct decision to preserve this important function.

One might think that a flexed knee contracture and a tight hamstring could be easily corrected by an orthopedic surgeon releasing or lengthening the hamstring. While it is likely that the hamstring tightness has contributed to the flexed knee contracture, over time the tight hamstring has also caused a tightening of the overall knee joint, including the knee capsule and knee ligaments that have both grown too long on the front and too short on the back of the knee. In addition, nerves and blood vessels will not have grown sufficiently long because they have been taking a "shortcut" to the lower leg over many years. Correcting a flexed knee contracture and a tight hamstring is not easy, but one method is addressed below.

Orthopedic surgery is addressed under the following headings:

- **Lower limb surgery**
- **Upper limb surgery**
- **Hip surgery**
- **Spine surgery**

Lower limb surgery

Children with spastic quadriplegia GMFCS level IV may walk short distances at home with a walker and adult supervision, but in adolescence and adulthood, they use a wheelchair in most settings. Lower limb surgery may be done to help the individual maintain their standing for transfers and limited walking in adolescence and adulthood, particularly if contractures and deformities from growth have contributed to a loss of previous skills. Extensive surgeries, however, may not be recommended as the risks may outweigh the benefits. Sustaining walking into adulthood may not be possible or practical.

Children with spastic quadriplegia GMFCS level V use a wheelchair for all mobility, and orthopedic surgery cannot help them to walk. In limited cases, orthopedic surgery may be considered to improve ability to tolerate using a stander, but the risks and magnitude of the surgery and subsequent rehabilitation may outweigh the benefits.

Lower limb surgery may be done to help with everyday function and comfort. For example, managing foot and ankle problems is important to allow for the use of orthoses and wearing shoes, and for the feet to be able to rest on the wheelchair footrests.[137]

A method that orthopedic surgeons commonly use to address knee flexion contracture is to surgically cut (osteotomy) the femur (thigh bone) just above the knee and remove a wedge of bone to allow the lower leg to more appropriately align with the upper leg. A metal plate and screws are inserted to maintain the alignment until the bone heals. This procedure is known as distal femoral extension osteotomy (DFEO). "Distal" refers to away from the center (i.e., the lower end of the femur), "femoral" refers to the femur, "extension" refers to straightening, and "osteotomy" refers to the surgical cutting of a bone.

> Due to Levi's poor reaction to lengthy surgeries, we have chosen to not put him through any "cosmetic" surgeries, as the benefits do not outweigh the costs. He does not seem in pain at all from having a knee contracture.

Upper limb surgery

Like lower limb surgery, upper limb orthopedic surgery to address an upper limb contracture may not be worth the risk or discomfort for children and adolescents with spastic quadriplegia if it will not result in improved function, comfort, or ability to complete the person's daily cares.

Hip surgery

Hip surgery for children with spastic quadriplegia GMFCS levels IV and V can be classified as **preventive, reconstructive,** and **salvage**.

Preventive surgery can be done when the migration percentage (MP) is less than 40. It is normally carried out at younger ages (three to six years).[137] It consists of soft tissue surgery for the hip adductors and hip flexors.[137]

Reconstructive surgery is needed if there is a high MP (greater than 40). It is normally carried out at somewhat older ages (five years or older).[137] It consists of three main components:[137]

- Soft tissue surgery—hip adductor release
- Bony surgery—femoral osteotomy
- Bony surgery—pelvic osteotomy

Hip surveillance must continue after either preventive or reconstructive surgery.[137]

Salvage surgery is needed when the hip can no longer be successfully reconstructed. Flattening of the femoral head, femoral head defects, or long-standing dislocation are the typical situations. (Hip dislocation is defined as MP over 90 and up to 100).[138] Salvage surgery is a major operation involving soft tissue and bone surgery.

The need for salvage surgery can be avoided by early hip surveillance and with appropriately timed preventive or reconstructive surgery. Salvage surgery outcomes are not as good as interventions at earlier stages.

Levi's hip dislocation was first surgically dealt with in 2015. They performed bilateral femoral derotations and lengthened his Achilles tendon. When puberty and rapid growth began in about 2019, his right hip again began to rotate out of the socket. In discussions with the surgeon, it was suggested that we consider a ventral dorsal rhizotomy prior to redoing the hips (otherwise the hip surgery would have to be redone a few years later). The rhizotomy would sever nearly all motor nerves and 80 percent of sensory nerves to the legs.

Levi had the ventral dorsal rhizotomy surgery in September 2020. While it did solve some of Levi's orthopedic issues, it caused an array of new issues, such as increased scoliosis and unwanted tone changes, and sped up our timeline for needing the spinal fusion surgery.

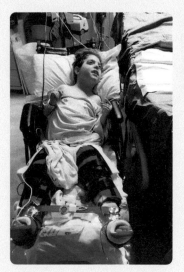 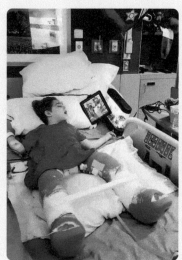

Levi after his hip surgery.

Spine surgery

As noted in section 2.5, scoliosis is common in individuals with spastic quadriplegia.

Spine surgery is an extensive procedure. It is understandable that providers and parents prefer to avoid it if the curve is smaller and its impact on function is less. However, if the curve is larger and significantly impacting function and respiratory health, or causing pain or positioning difficulty, there is value in doing spine surgery for the overall comfort and health of the individual.

For individuals with CP, the following are indications for spine surgery to address scoliosis.[223,224]

- Cobb angle greater than 40 to 50 degrees that is either progressive (becoming larger over time) or interfering with sitting

- Spinal orthosis being intolerable or not correcting sitting challenges
- Individual experiencing pain, respiratory dysfunction, or abdominal issues clearly related to the spine or spinal orthosis
- Age greater than 10 years
- Adequate hip ROM to enable proper seating after surgery
- Stable nutritional and medical status

The most common type of spine surgery in individuals with CP is spinal fusion. During this procedure, two or more vertebrae in the spine are fused together (joined into one). A spinal fusion can be performed through the patient's back (posterior spinal fusion), the patient's front (anterior spinal fusion), or a combination of both approaches. Posterior spinal fusion is by far the most common. Implants are attached to the spinal bone (screws are most common), and a metal rod is then connected to them to straighten the spine and hold it in the straight position.

There are three main goals for spinal fusion in adolescents or young adults with CP: improve the spinal curve, achieve a durable stable new spinal shape, and ensure a safe and tolerable surgery.[224] Improvement of the spinal curve does not mean reducing the Cobb angle to an absolute minimum, but instead achieving a level pelvis with a well-centered or balanced trunk.[224]

Studies show that spinal fusion positively impacts health-related quality of life in individuals with CP GMFCS levels IV and V.[225,226] Caregivers ranked spinal fusion as the second-most beneficial intervention for individuals with CP GMFCS IV and V.[227] The only intervention ranked above it was insertion of a gastrostomy tube (see section 3.3). As with all surgery, the benefits of spinal fusion may not outweigh the risks for individuals with spastic quadriplegia who have severe medical challenges.

More information on the management of scoliosis in individuals with spastic quadriplegia is included in **Useful web resources**.

Levi had frequent spine X-rays throughout his first eight years. Around his ninth birthday, an X-ray noted a spine curvature, and we were sent to a spine specialist. X-rays done every six months showed the spine remaining relatively stable—around a 25- to 30-degree curvature. But after the ventral dorsal rhizotomy and the onset of puberty, curvature increased, and we opted to intervene with spinal rod placement.[*] That surgery was the most difficult for him to recover from as he had trouble with wound healing and postoperative lung function.

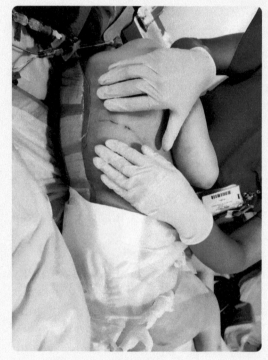

Levi after his spine surgery.

---

[*] Spinal fusion.

Key points Chapter 5

- The overall goal of managing musculoskeletal health (i.e., orthopedic care) is to prevent and treat musculoskeletal problems that may interfere with function, ease of daily cares, and comfort now or in the future to allow the individual to participate as fully as possible in life.
- Managing musculoskeletal health includes tone reduction, musculoskeletal surveillance, and orthopedic surgery.
- For musculoskeletal treatments, having a multidisciplinary team and shared goal-setting between the individual with their family and medical professionals is very important, with everyone considering and weighing the benefits and risks of the intervention against those of not proceeding with the surgery.
- Treatment of high tone includes the daily home stretching program, casting, and/or orthotics, oral or enteral medications, injectable medications (BoNT-A and phenol), and neurosurgery (including intrathecal baclofen, ventral dorsal rhizotomy, and deep brain stimulation).
- Musculoskeletal surveillance involves regular monitoring and assessment of musculoskeletal development and function. It includes surveillance of lower and upper limb range of motion, hip displacement, spinal curvature, and bone health.
- Orthopedic surgery includes surgery on the lower limb, upper limb, hip, and spine.
- Hip surgery can be classified as preventive, reconstructive, and salvage. The need for salvage surgery can be avoided by early hip surveillance and with appropriately timed preventive or reconstructive surgery. Salvage surgery outcomes are not as good as interventions at earlier stages.
- Both neurosurgery and orthopedic surgery are big undertakings for individuals with spastic quadriplegia as their general health status is often more difficult to maintain and the risk of complication is higher. Preoperative general health status must be assessed and optimized and there must be a focus on excellent postoperative care.

Chapter 6

Increasing participation

Introduction

> Disability is not a tragedy; discrimination and
> lack of accessibility are the real tragedies.
>
> Tom Shakespeare

Spastic quadriplegia is a complex form of CP, and as we have seen across this book, it significantly impacts many body systems. Given the interconnectedness of different levels of functioning as shown in the ICF (see Figure 1.8.1), problems at the body functions and structure, and activity levels have a big impact on participation. This section addresses level 4 considerations—increasing participation for individuals with spastic quadriplegia.

USEFUL WEB RESOURCES

Cognition and intelligence

You are not a drop in the ocean.
You are the entire ocean in a drop.
Rumi

Cognition can be defined as the mental action or process of acquiring knowledge and understanding through thought, experience, and the senses. **Intelligence** can be defined as the overall mental capacity to understand complex ideas, adapt to the environment, learn from experience, engage in reasoning, and overcome obstacles. **Intellectual disability** can be defined as[228] problems with general mental abilities that affect areas of intellectual functioning (such as learning, problem-solving, judgment) and adaptive functioning (activities of daily life such as communication and independent living).

The diagnosis of intellectual disability is typically made during the developmental period (i.e., during childhood or adolescence) when problems in intellectual functioning and adaptive functioning become apparent.[229] Each is measured as follows:

- **Intellectual functioning** may be measured using standardized testing, often yielding an intelligence quotient (IQ). In a typical population, the broad average range of IQ scores is between 85 and 115. An IQ score of 70 or below suggests intellectual challenges.[229]
- **Adaptive functioning** may be measured using various standardized tests and scales that assess skills such as communication, social interaction, independence, and functioning in educational or vocational settings. These assessments provide normed scores, allowing professionals to gauge the individual's abilities compared with peers.

The diagnosis of intellectual disability is then made based on scores of intellectual functioning (IQ typically below 70), adaptive functioning, and clinical history. Additional information gained from neuropsychological testing (see below) is also considered.

Recall from section 2.1 that an Australian study found 42 percent of children age five with spastic quadriplegia (all GMFCS levels) had moderate or severe intellectual challenges (moderate: IQ 35 to 49; severe: IQ less than 35), while a further 32 percent had mild or some impairment (IQ 50 to 69).[80] The prevalence and severity of associated problems were found to correlate with GMFCS level.[80]

Indeed, as the authors of the Australian study noted, it can be challenging to accurately measure intellectual function in children with severe motor, visual, and/or communication problems. Testing may need to be modified as appropriate and results interpreted carefully.[180] In addition, consideration of mental or behavioral health needs within the context of testing is important. An accurate assessment of a child that is particularly anxious or behaviorally acting out may not be recommended until management of the anxiety or other mental health or behavioral health symptoms is achieved. It is important that the child's intellectual ability not be underestimated.

Neuropsychological testing can be very helpful here. Neuropsychology is the study of the relationship of the brain and behaviors and how they impact each other. The brain impacts behaviors that we see, and in turn, behaviors allow us to examine how the brain functions.[230] The testing of brain functions and behaviors is broadly referred to as neuropsychological testing. It includes testing, for example, intelligence, language, visuospatial function (ability to recognize, interpret, and mentally manipulate visual information and spatial relationships), executive function (planning, organization, working memory, self-regulation, flexible thinking, making choices, and task initiation), attention, memory, and processing speed. These areas frequently work in collaboration for efficient cognitive functioning.

Early screening for intellectual functioning and identification of intellectual disability can help guide educational planning and supportive intervention services for the child to maximize their intellectual function and ensure the best possible outcomes. As the child grows, additional areas of concern may become more apparent, especially as task demands increase with age, highlighting the need for follow-up evaluations to ensure appropriate services at each stage of development.

In the US, when children with CP enter the school system around their third birthday, an individualized education plan (IEP) may be created through a process involving parents and caregivers, the special education team, school therapists, and the school psychologist.[180] This plan is updated annually and reevaluated at least every three years. Appropriate supports (e.g., adapted education, therapy services, assistive technology) frequently need to be put in place to maximize the educational growth of the child.[180] Some teachers have specialized training, for example, for teaching children with visual or hearing impairment.

Targeted strategies can help improve cognitive participation for children with CP. These include activities to address skills such as attention, communication, processing and comprehension, memory, problem-solving, and executive functioning. Some of these skills are also needed to successfully use adaptive communication devices. The following are some ideas for more activities at home to facilitate these skills:

- **Playing board games:** For attention, taking turns, following directions, working memory, planning, strategizing, communication skills, and developmental skills (including counting, vocabulary, and categorization)
- **Karaoke or songs that require gestures:** For articulation, memory and/or reading skills, breath support/control for speech production, volume and fine motor skills, developing signs to augment communication, and cognitive development

- **Reading and listening to audiobooks:** For vocabulary development, communication skills, memory, comprehension, and processing skills
- **Joining social groups:** For example, scouts, church groups to encourage social communication, mental flexibility, attention, and play skills
- **Playing word games:** For example, "I spy" while in the car to work on vocabulary, descriptive language, speech production, and memorization
- **Making up stories:** Having the child pick characters, actions, and settings to allow and encourage them to make choices.
- **Playing object or picture identification games:** Having the child verbally name or point or even look at the item.

Many other strategies are used in occupational therapy and speech and language pathology.

Levi was born with neurotypical brain function. The damage came during his ostomy takedown surgery, with the brain scan that followed showing the majority of damage to his white matter. His gray matter was normal, leading us to believe he has fairly normal cognition but with no way to communicate this sufficiently. Some things that lead us to believe his cognition is typical include his ability to manipulate the people around him to do what he wants, and his ability to laugh when one of his siblings gets in trouble. He even teases them when they are watching him by crying loudly until they come to check on him, then laughing when they get to him. He is a sassy and spunky dude!

IQ tests require motor skills and language to complete. Children with spastic quadriplegia have limited or seriously impacted purposeful fine motor, gross motor, and oral language skills. But just because these areas are limited does not mean their cognition is limited! There is no IQ test today that can test cognition without motor skills or oral language skills impacting the score. That's why I have turned down IQ tests for Levi and refused to allow him to be labeled as cognitively delayed.

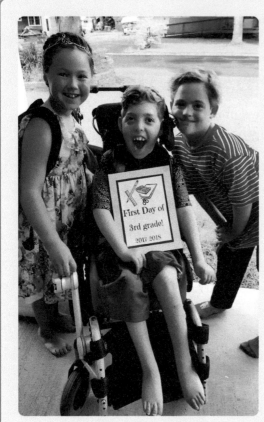

Ana, Levi, and Cam on their first day of third grade.

Mental and behavioral health

In the midst of Winter, I found there was,
within me, an invincible Summer.

Albert Camus

Mental health has been defined as "a state of mental well-being that enables people to cope with the stresses of life, realize their abilities, learn well and work well, and contribute to their community."[231] While mental and behavioral health are closely related, they are different. No formal definition was found, but behavioral health has more to do with how people react in a situation—two people in the same situation may react in very different ways. Mental health has more to do with thoughts and emotions. Mental and behavioral health strongly contribute to quality of life.

Mental health

Individuals with spastic quadriplegia are at risk for mental health challenges. A number of studies have reported a higher level of mental health symptoms and disorders among children and adolescents with CP.[232,233,234]

- A Norwegian study of young children, 88 percent with spastic CP GMFCS levels I to IV, found that 57 percent had a mental health condition, with attention deficit disorder (ADD) and attention deficit hyperactivity disorder (ADHD) the most common.[232] Children with communication problems were at a higher risk of having a mental health condition.[232]
- A systematic review and meta-analysis[*] concluded that children with CP and intellectual disability have a higher risk of mental health symptoms.[233]
- A Danish study reported that the prevalence of mental health disorders was significantly higher in children and adolescents with CP (22 percent) compared with peers (6 percent).[234]
- Data from the US shows that children with CP are more likely to have an autism spectrum disorder than children in the typical population (7 percent versus 1 percent).[235]

Behavioral health

Novak and colleagues reported that one in four children with CP have a behavior disorder. However, they note that children with CP and severe physical disability are less likely to have behavioral problems than those with milder physical disability.[174]

Behavioral challenges may present in a variety of daily tasks such as sleeping, feeding, and toileting, and these behaviors can present as aggression, self-injury, disruption, tantrums, and noncompliance.[236] In nonverbal individuals, behavioral outbursts can be due to pain, hunger, fatigue, or change in routine, among other causes. Ruling out physical reasons for behaviors is an appropriate first step in behavioral management.[237]

---

[*] A systematic review summarizes the results of several scientific studies on the same topic. It can be qualitative (descriptive) or quantitative (numerical). The quantitative approach is called a meta-analysis.

Children with CP often have sensory problems. For example, they may over- or underreact to tactile information. Overreaction can result in irritability from being touched or from wearing certain clothing. Underreaction can include a lack of response to painful injuries.[236]

Levi does not seem to have any behavioral challenges. However, he is a master manipulator and can get most people to do what he wants them to do pretty easily!

Evaluations for mental and behavioral health should be incorporated into multidisciplinary team assessments and appropriate treatments should be prescribed. Treatments for mental and behavioral health disorders may include psychotherapy, medications, and behavioral therapy. Parenting programs that help parents manage challenging behavior may be of help. There is evidence supporting the Stepping Stones Triple P program for improving child behavior and reducing parental stress.[14] This program, specifically for parents of preadolescent children who have a disability, is available online and is included in **Useful web resources.**

Puberty and sexual expression

As we let our own light shine, we unconsciously give other people permission to do the same.

Nelson Mandela

A study found that sexual maturation in children with CP GMFCS levels III to V differs from that of children in the general population.[238] Specifically, compared with white children in the general population, puberty begins earlier but ends later in white children with CP, and menarche (first occurrence of menstruation) occurs later in white girls with CP.[238] The timing of menarche is related to skeletal maturation (girls are considered skeletally mature when they reach final adult height, approximately two years after menarche) and this is important in orthopedic surgery planning.[239]

The onset of menstruation can present challenges for females with spastic quadriplegia, including hygiene and pain. Hygiene during menstruation may mean more frequent transfers and changing. Pain related to menstruation may worsen tone.[240] For some, hormonal therapy can be an appropriate option to manage menstruation.[240] Females with epilepsy may also experience changes in seizure control due to hormonal fluctuations related to menstruation.[241] Birth control and protection against sexually transmitted infections should also be provided as appropriate. Some antiseizure medications are known to interact with hormonal birth control, making the birth control ineffective and leading to unplanned pregnancy.[242]

Females with disabilities are at a higher risk of sexual abuse than those in the general population.[240] Education about sexual abuse, indicators of abuse, and referrals for support services should be provided for all individuals with spastic quadriplegia (i.e., all genders) and their family members.

Adolescents with spastic quadriplegia have the right to sexual expression and should receive appropriate support and education in this area from a multidisciplinary team that includes health care providers, psychologists, and counselors. Health care providers should ask questions about these issues as the individual continues to mature, but if this is not the case, advocating for discussion on these topics is important. Addressing concerns about body image, self-esteem, and relationships is also important. Sexual function and intimacy may require adaptive positioning and equipment that occupational therapists, physical therapists, and recreational therapists may help with.

Community integration

The power of community to create health is far
greater than any physician, clinic or hospital.

Mark Hyman

Maximizing activity and participation requires a comprehensive management approach. If challenges are addressed, individuals with spastic quadriplegia can be supported to actively participate in society, promoting their overall well-being and quality of life as well as enhancing the lives of others. Strategies for community integration can include accessible transportation, inclusive recreational activities, educational accommodations, and promoting peer relationships. Providing assistive technology and environmental modifications can enhance participation in community settings. Collaboration between medical professionals, educators, social workers, and community organizations is crucial to facilitate integration of children and adolescents with spastic quadriplegia into their communities.

The F-words (see section 1.8 and Figure 1.8.2) encourage families to play to strengths, focusing on what the individual can do rather than what they can't do. Recall that the F-word "functioning" is about activity: "I might do things differently, but I CAN do them. How I do it is not important. Please let me try!" The famous writer and artist Christy Brown who had spastic quadriplegia is an example of applying this sentiment. He wrote and painted with his left foot.

This strengths-based approach is very important throughout childhood and adolescence, as well as later in adulthood (addressed in Chapter 9). Achieving function may require a lot of assistance and adaptation, whether for mobility, communication, eating, or drinking. The "how" is not important; the participation is.

Physical medicine and rehabilitation (PM&R), a branch of medicine, aims to bridge the gap between problems at the level of body functions and structure and the level of participation, helping individuals overcome barriers. While advancements in medical science may offer more solutions in the future, and while we continue to advocate for progress, it is crucial not to wait until then. By adopting a strengths-based approach and emphasizing comprehensive care now, we can support individuals with spastic quadriplegia and empower them to live fulfilling lives.

> Levi has participated in many community activities such as downhill skiing and swimming lessons. We are active travelers and frequently go out of state for vacations. Levi adores roller-coasters and other rides.

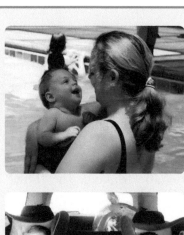
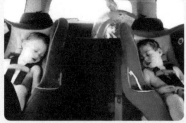
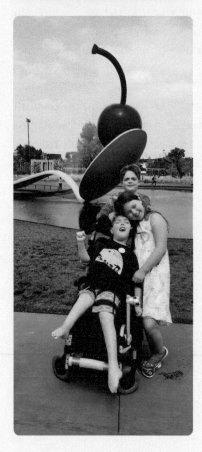
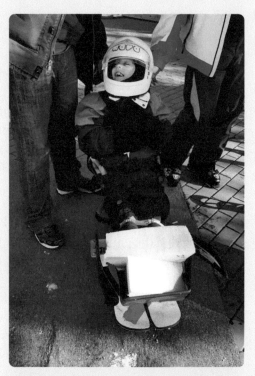
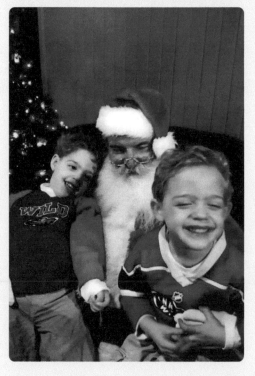

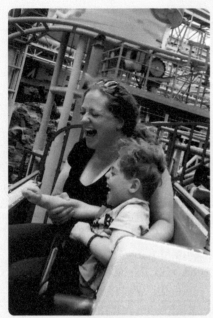
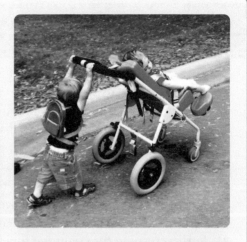
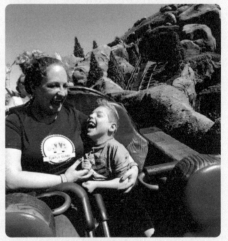
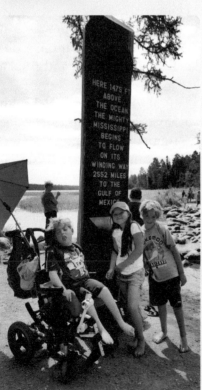
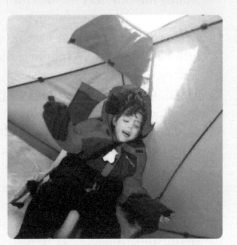

Ana, Cam, and Levi on various family outings with Aunt Jess.

Key points Chapter 6

- Many individuals with spastic quadriplegia GMFCS levels IV and V have intellectual challenges ranging from mild to severe.
- The diagnosis of intellectual disability is typically made during childhood or adolescence when problems in intellectual functioning and adaptive functioning become apparent.
- Neuropsychological testing helps to evaluate broad areas of cognitive function; for example, intelligence, language, visuospatial function, executive function, attention, memory, and processing speed.
- Early screening for cognitive functioning and identification of intellectual disability can help guide educational planning and supportive intervention services for the child to maximize their cognitive function. Appropriate supports (e.g., adapted education, therapy services, and assistive technology) frequently need to be put in place to maximize the educational growth of the child.
- It can be challenging to accurately measure cognitive function in children with severe motor, visual, and/or communication problems. Testing may need to be modified as appropriate and results interpreted carefully.
- Children with spastic quadriplegia are at risk for mental health problems. In nonverbal individuals, behavioral outbursts can be due to pain, hunger, fatigue, or change in routine, among other causes. Ruling out physical reasons for behaviors is an appropriate first step in behavioral management.
- Evaluations for mental and behavioral health should be incorporated into multidisciplinary team assessments and appropriate treatments prescribed.
- The onset of menstruation can present challenges for females with spastic quadriplegia, including hygiene and pain.
- Adolescents with spastic quadriplegia have the right to sexual expression and should receive appropriate support and education in this area from a multidisciplinary team, including health care providers, psychologists, and counselors.
- Maximizing activity and participation requires a comprehensive management approach. By addressing challenges, individuals with spastic quadriplegia can be supported to actively participate in society, promoting their overall well-being and quality of life.

- Strategies for community integration can include accessible transportation, inclusive recreational activities, educational accommodations, and promoting peer relationships.

Chapter 7

Alternative and complementary treatments

> It is possible in medicine, even when you intend to do good,
> to do harm instead. That is why science thrives on actively
> encouraging criticism rather than stifling it.
> **Richard Dawkins**

Alternative (as a substitute) and complementary (in addition to) treatments are treatments that are not part of current standard conventional medical or rehabilitation treatments and care.[243]

Parents want only the best for their children, and for a number of reasons they may consider alternative and complementary treatments. These reasons can include:

- Hearing about a treatment option in the media (Internet, radio, TV, newspapers, magazines) or from well-meaning family and friends
- Wanting to try all treatment options in case the one they haven't tried is the one that works
- Wanting to complement or increase the effectiveness of present treatment
- Wanting to relieve symptoms (such as pain)
- Believing their child can do better

Often, alternative and complementary treatments are expensive. If the parent-professional relationship is good, parents should be able to discuss them with the medical professionals who treat their child. Both parents and professionals should be guided by the best research evidence available, which is the very principle that has guided the writing of this book.

Table 7.1 lists a number of common alternative and complementary treatments.

Table 7.1 Alternative and complementary treatments

TREATMENT	DESCRIPTION	EVIDENCE (OR LACK OF) SUPPORTING TREATMENT IN CP
Hyperbaric oxygen	The person inhales 100 percent oxygen in a pressurized hyperbaric chamber. The theory behind its use in CP is that there are inactive cells among the damaged brain cells that have the potential to recover.	**Strong recommendation against its use for all purposes.**[14]
Massage	Involves applying pressure to muscles, generally using the hands, to relieve pain and tension.	**Strong recommendation for improved passage of stool.**[14] Probably effective for other purposes.[14]
Osteopathy (including cranial sacral osteopathy)	Treatment through the manipulation and massage of skeleton and muscles. Cranial sacral osteopathy focuses on the cranium (bones of the skull) and sacrum (the five fused vertebrae that connect the spine to the pelvis).	**Strong recommendation against its use for improved gross motor function.**[14] Probably effective for reduced constipation and improved sleep.[14]
Acupuncture	Thin needles are inserted into the skin at specific points.	Probably effective for improved gross motor function and reduced spasticity.[14]
Reflexology	Massage based on the theory that there are reflex points on the feet, hands, and head linked to every part of the body.	Probably effective for reduced spasticity, improved gross motor function, and reduced constipation.[14]

Novak and colleagues' summary of the state of the evidence as of 2019 for interventions for children with CP (including further alternative and complementary treatments),[14] is included in **Useful web resources.**

A Canadian study looked at the extent to which adolescents with CP across all five GMFCS levels had used alternative and complementary treatments in the previous year. The most commonly used services were massage (15 percent), hyperbaric oxygen (10 percent), and osteopathy (6 percent), but most of those surveyed (73 percent) did not currently use any.[243]

Graham noted that many parents delay or refuse conventional treatments because they have unrealistic expectations of other unproven treatments. For example, although Australia has an efficient hip surveillance program, the most common cause of a dislocated hip in a child with CP is delayed intervention because they have heard that stem cell treatment* may cure the child.[244]

Parents cannot afford to abandon conventional treatments with their evidence base for any unproven treatment, nor should they delay care that is currently available for their child, anticipating a better option is "around the corner." As treatments are studied and when they are identified as potentially helpful, good physicians will be aware of the developing research and will share with families if any new options are on the horizon.

---

* An alternative treatment that may potentially replace damaged nerve cells and support remaining ones in the brain.

Chapter 8

Transition to adulthood

At the end of adolescence, health care for the individual with spastic quadriplegia usually changes from pediatric to adult services, and this can be a daunting change. It can be a big challenge for an adolescent to lose the services from professionals that they have effectively grown up with.

Health care transition is defined as the planned process and skill-building to empower adolescents and their families to navigate and integrate into an adult model of health care. It is more than simply changing medical professionals (termed "transfer").

Pediatric services for CP care are usually much better resourced than adult services and are more proactive in following up with the individual. With adult services for CP care, it is usually up to the individual and family to do more proactive service procuring. Adult services are often much more reactionary rather than proactive.

Transition lasts well over a decade, starting at approximately 12 years old and involves three steps: preparing, transferring, and integrating into adult services. That is, just because a file has been transferred does not mean that the individual has successfully integrated into an adult service provider.

Transition doesn't just involve health care; it also involves other areas such as education, finance, insurance coverage, and guardianship planning. Figure 8.1 is a comprehensive look at some important transition questions: Where will I live? Who is my care team? How will I pay for things? What will I do?

It is very important that the individual with CP be involved in the discussion and planning of their transition to adulthood insofar as possible.

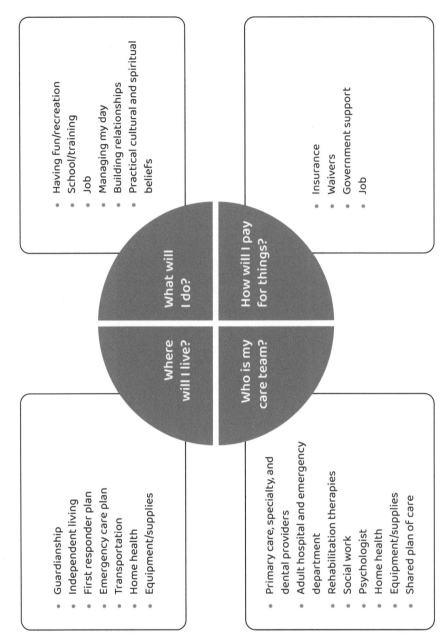

Figure 8.1 Some important transition questions.

Figure 8.2 shows a typical form that can be used for preparing an individual for transition to adult services.

Transition Readiness Assessment Questionnaire (TRAQ)

Patient Name: _____ Date of Birth: ___/___/___ Today's Date ___/___/___ (MRN#_____)

Directions to Youth and Young Adults: Please check the box that best describes _your_ skill level in the following areas that are important for transition to adult health care. There is no right or wrong answer and your answers will remain confidential and private.
Directions to Caregivers/Parents: If your youth or young adult is unable to complete the tasks below on their own, please check the box that best describes _your_ skill level. **Check here** if you are a parent/caregiver completing this form. ☐

	No, I do not know how	No, but I want to learn	No, but I am learning to do this	Yes, I have started doing this	Yes, I always do this when I need to
Managing Medications					
1. Do you fill a prescription if you need to?					
2. Do you know what to do if you are having a bad reaction to your medications?					
3. Do you reorder medications before they run out?					
4. Do you explain any medications (name and dose) you are taking to healthcare providers?					
5. Do you speak with the pharmacist about drug interactions or other concerns related to your medications?					
Appointment Keeping					
6. Do you call the doctor's office to make an appointment?					
7. Do you follow-up on referrals for tests or check-ups or labs?					
8. Do you arrange for your ride to medical appointments?					
9. Do you call the doctor about unusual changes in your health (for example: allergic reactions)?					
Tracking Health Issues					
10. Do you fill out the medical history form, including a list of your allergies?					
11. Do you keep a calendar or list of medical and other appointments?					
12. Do you tell the doctor or nurse what you are feeling?					
13. Do you contact the doctor when you have a health concern?					
14. Do you make or help make medical decisions pertaining to your health?					
15. Do you attend your medical appointment or part of your appointment by yourself?					
Talking with Providers					
16. Do you ask questions of your nurse or doctor about your health or health care?					
17. Do you answer questions that are asked by the doctor, nurse, or clinic staff?					
18. Do you ask your doctor or nurse to explain things more clearly if you do not understand their instructions to you?					
19. Do you tell the doctor or nurse whether you followed their advice or recommendations?					
20. Do you explain your health history to your healthcare providers (including past surgeries, allergies, and medications)?					

Please circle how you feel about the following statements

	Not at all important	Not too important	Somewhat important	Important	Very Important
How important is it to you to manage your own health care?	1	2	3	4	5
How confident do you feel about your ability to manage your own health care?	1	2	3	4	5

© Wood, Reiss, & Livingood, McBee, Johnson, 2020

Figure 8.2 Transition Readiness Assessment Questionnaire. Reproduced with kind permission from Dr. David L. Wood.

We saw in Chapter 1 that interdependence rather than independence may be the better goal. In life, all of us are interdependent to varying degrees, no one is an island.

Involving individuals with severe disabilities in decision-making about their future to the greatest extent possible is not just a matter of basic human rights, it is a crucial step toward empowerment and inclusivity. By actively listening to their thoughts, views, and expectations, we honor their autonomy and recognize their unique perspectives. Each person's journey is deeply personal, and by incorporating their input, we can tailor support and services to meet their specific needs and aspirations. Emphasizing their voice in decision-making fosters a sense of dignity, self-worth, and belonging, allowing them to lead fulfilling lives with a sense of agency and purpose. In creating a society where their opinions are valued, we embrace the richness of diversity and create a more compassionate, equitable, and truly inclusive community. *Independent of cognitive level*, young adults with disabilities who demonstrate increased levels of self-determination (the ability to act as their own primary decision maker) have been found to fare better across multiple life categories, including employment, access to health care and other benefits, financial independence, and independent living.[245]

Another point to consider is how transition will affect adult siblings. They may anticipate having to take on guardianship responsibilities in the future when parents are no longer able to fulfill that role, and they may make life choices on that basis; for example, choosing to live closer to the family home.

Got Transition is a US federally funded national resource center for health care transition. Its aim is to improve transition from pediatric to adult health care through the use of evidence-driven strategies for health care professionals, youth, young adults, and their families. The website has a lot of useful guidance.

In its *Lifespan Journal Digest*, the American Academy of Cerebral Palsy and Developmental Medicine routinely spotlight recent studies focused on lifespan issues, including the transition to adult care and aging with a disability.

Links to both are included in **Useful web resources**.

Having a child with a disability puts extra strain on a marriage. I wish I had known that when I had my twins in 2009. Perhaps I would have prioritized my self-care, communication, and relationship with my then husband. Though had I done that, I never would have met my current husband or had the beautiful opportunity to raise three same-age kids. I wouldn't change how my path turned out, though I do now remind couples who have special needs children to prioritize their relationship.

Levi is now blessed with not only an identical twin but an amazing same-age bonus stepsister as well. Both of Levi's siblings have experienced the stress and trauma of having a brother with special needs. They have watched him go through dozens of surgeries and countless hospitalizations. They have seen Levi receive vast amounts of attention (rightly so), but their young minds were not able to put context to the situation. Cameron, Levi's twin, did attend special therapy for siblings of special needs when he was about five years old, and his sister has attended therapy to support her as well.

Levi's sister has always had a caretaking role with him, though she herself has type 1 diabetes. When she was only three, she showed interest in tube-feeding Levi, and she has always ensured he was included in any activities we did as a family. She hand-over-hand colored and painted with him and would soothe him when he was upset. Levi's twin is a little more anxious in his relationship with his brother, though now at 14 he acts as Levi's bus aid and is constantly responding to Levi's whining for a new episode of his favorite shows. We have done our best to spend time with each of our children individually, and we ensure that each gets what they need. We have a lot of fun together going on adventures and include Levi in all that we do.

We recognize that Levi's siblings have been impacted by Levi having such extensive medical needs. They both have medical trauma from this, and they both have developed anxiety disorders (though not necessarily solely from having a sibling with special needs, it most certainly adds to the condition).

Parents need to take care of themselves in order to effectively care for their child and family. Neglecting their own well-being can have detrimental effects on mental and physical health.

My husband and I decided that we had to get fit and strong in order to be able to properly care for Levi as long as possible. In 2017, we joined the YMCA, lost 50 pounds each, and began weekly strength training. By putting our health first and doing it together, we stayed motivated, grew in our relationship, and were better able to lift Levi. We are still strength training and running together, and we prioritize our physical and mental health. We hope to teach this self-care to Levi's siblings as well.

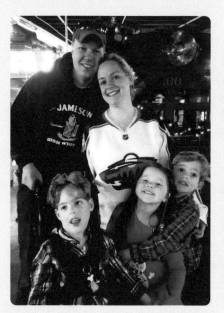
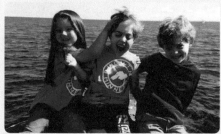
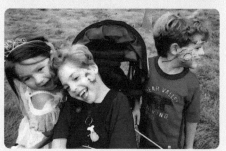

Left: Bonus dad, David, with Kate, Levi, Ana, and Cam; Top right: Ana, Levi, and Cam; Botton Right: Ana, Levi, and Cam.

USEFUL WEB RESOURCES

Chapter 9

Adulthood

Introduction

With mirth and laughter let old wrinkles come.

William Shakespeare

CP is diagnosed in childhood and is a lifelong condition. It is often thought of as a children's condition, but it is not. Having a severe form of CP is not easy for the individual or their family. The severity of problems affects life expectancy; however, over the past three decades, data from California has shown that there have been significant improvements in the survival of children with CP and severe disability.[246] Over that time frame, treatment and care for children with severe CP has improved, with added focus on areas including the management of seizures, nutrition, scoliosis, infections, and respiratory issues.[247]

The World Health Organization (WHO) defines an adult as a person older than 19 years of age.[248] But what does being an adult really mean? While everybody's path in life is different, one description of being an adult includes the following accomplishments.[249]

Completing formal education, entering the labor force, living independently, having romantic relationships and sexual experiences, getting married and having children, establishing peer and family relationships, participating in recreation/leisure, driving a car, and enjoying group social encounters.

The extent to which an individual with spastic quadriplegia GMFCS levels IV and V accomplishes any or all of these depends on the severity of their impairments and their support system. We saw in section 2.1 that two in five children with spastic quadriplegia have moderate to severe intellectual problems. Many, but not all, adults with spastic quadriplegia will likely need supported living arrangements and support with decision-making.

As a person with spastic quadriplegia reaches adulthood and skeletal growth has ceased, a certain stabilization of the musculoskeletal aspects of the condition occurs. The rate of change of the condition is slower in adulthood, assuming the adult remains physically active. People with spastic quadriplegia may, however, develop secondary conditions in adulthood. Some of these are consistent with typical aging, but some may be unique. Each may influence body systems in more complex ways because of the interactions with CP itself.

The Centers for Disease Control and Prevention (CDC) explain secondary conditions as follows:[250]

As a result of having a specific type of disability, such as a spinal cord injury ... other physical or mental health conditions can occur. Some of these other health conditions are also called secondary conditions ...

The specific secondary conditions that may develop depend on the primary condition. For example, eye problems are secondary conditions that may develop from having diabetes; osteoarthritis is a secondary condition that may develop from having spastic quadriplegia. This chapter addresses the secondary conditions associated with spastic quadriplegia. Note that the secondary conditions referred to here are general health conditions and separate from the secondary musculoskeletal problems that develop as a result of the primary brain injury in CP addressed in section 2.5.

The development of secondary conditions is not inevitable. Good management can help prevent or minimize their development. Though they are addressed in this chapter on adulthood, some secondary conditions may appear earlier in life.

In childhood and adolescence, growth is a challenge for the person with spastic quadriplegia. In adulthood, typical aging becomes a challenge. Though there are far more adults than children with CP, most of the efforts of health care professionals are directed at children and adolescents. Meeting the needs of young people with CP is absolutely essential, but given that CP is a lifelong condition and further issues may arise with age, the medical establishment must better address the lack of service provision for adults with CP. To that end, currently, a clinical practice guideline for adults with CP is being developed. Once published, the guideline will, hopefully, pave the way for better service provision for adults with CP.

As well, much of the limited research in CP to date has focused on children, and as we saw in section 2.2, more severe forms of CP are less represented in research studies. An analysis of National Institutes of Health (NIH)* funding for CP research from 2001 to 2013 found that only 4 percent of available funding went toward studies of CP in adulthood.[251] As well, as was noted earlier in this book, funding generally for CP research is very low relative to the prevalence of the condition and its impact across the life span.

While research on CP in adulthood is considerably less than in childhood, it has been growing over time, as shown by the increase in the annual number of studies from a search using the terms "cerebral palsy" and "adult." See Figure 9.1.1.

---

* The NIH is the primary US body responsible for health research.

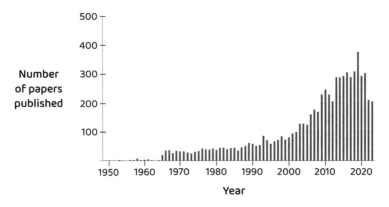

Figure 9.1.1 Number of studies on CP in adulthood per year (PubMed).*

More research is needed to fully understand how CP changes in adulthood and what can be done to prevent or minimize the problems that arise as adults with CP age. Because "adults" range in age from 19 to 80-plus years, they are not a homogenous group. It is necessary to have a better sense of how health care challenges evolve across the decades. Longitudinal research studies for adults with CP as they age would offer valuable information. A 2008 workshop to define the challenges of treating and preventing secondary conditions in adults with CP concluded with this very worthy goal:[252]

> *The same sense of responsibility and compassion that motivated the research that led to such advances as increasing the survival rates of very low birth weight infants must now be applied to developing the best means of caring for children with CP as they reach adulthood ... The medical and research communities have helped these individuals survive. It is now our responsibility to help them thrive and live productive lives, as uninhibited as possible by the chronic pain and secondary conditions associated with CP.*

USEFUL WEB RESOURCES

---

* A free online database of medical and life sciences research articles.

Aging in the typical population

> In a gentle way, you can shake the world.
> Mahatma Gandhi

The *Oxford English Dictionary* defines aging as "the process of growing old." But that doesn't give us much information. The fact that decline occurs with age is obvious from observing those around us. Before addressing aging in adults with CP, let us first look at aging in the typical population.

Examples of the decline that may occur with age include sarcopenia (loss of skeletal muscle mass and strength), joint pain, osteoarthritis, osteoporosis, falls, and low-trauma fractures (easily acquired bone breaks). Many conditions become more prevalent as people age, including cardiovascular disease, cancer, respiratory disease, and diabetes. These conditions are termed "noncommunicable diseases" (NCDs).

Some of the above can be considered part of "normal" aging (e.g., sarcopenia), but most are diagnosable medical conditions. Diagnosable medical conditions occur in the typical population, but they are not "normal." This section addresses sarcopenia and NCDs in more detail.

Sarcopenia

Sarcopenia is the loss of skeletal muscle mass and strength.[253] Typically developing adults achieve peak muscle mass by their early 40s, which progressively declines and results in as much as 50 percent loss by the time they are in their 80s. As we saw earlier, muscle strength is related to muscle size. Losing muscle mass has consequences for maintaining the level of function we need to carry out activities of daily living as we age; for example, even just getting up from a chair. By performing simple muscle strengthening exercises, adults can offset the natural loss of muscle mass that commonly occurs with age.

Protein is required for muscle growth. Older people are less efficient than younger people at extracting protein from food, which means older people need to be especially vigilant about meeting their daily protein needs.[254]

Noncommunicable diseases

A noncommunicable disease (NCD) is a medical condition not caused by an infectious agent.[*] NCDs, also known as chronic diseases, tend to be of long duration. The World Health Organization reported that NCDs are the cause of over three-quarters of all deaths globally. The following four conditions account for over 80 percent of all deaths due to NCDs.[255]

- Cardiovascular disease (e.g., heart attack and stroke)
- Cancer
- Respiratory disease (e.g., chronic obstructive pulmonary disease and asthma)
- Diabetes

In section 1.3, we examined the difference between causes and risk factors. NCDs share four behavioral risk factors:[255]

- Tobacco use
- Physical inactivity

---

[*] A communicable disease is caused by an infectious agent such as a bacterium or virus.

- Unhealthy diet
- Excess alcohol consumption

People have control over each of these risk factors—they are lifestyle choices. However, it is important to acknowledge that socioeconomic factors can adversely affect nutrition and health. Very often, multiple combinations may be present, such as an unhealthy diet combined with physical inactivity.

Cardiometabolic risk factors ("cardio" refers to heart and "metabolic," refers to the process the body uses to turn food into energy) include:

- High levels of blood cholesterol (a type of fat in the blood)
- High levels of triglycerides (another type of fat in the blood)
- High blood pressure (also termed "hypertension")
- Insulin resistance[*] or diabetes
- Being overweight or obese[†]
- Metabolic syndrome (a person is diagnosed with metabolic syndrome if they have at least three of the five risk factors above)
- High levels of C-reactive protein (a protein in the blood; high levels are a sign of inflammation in the body)

In addition to good lifestyle choices, regular health checks with a primary care provider are important for managing our health as we age. A primary care provider will check many of the above risk factors. Most developed countries also have screening programs for many cancers, such as breast and colon cancer. Appropriate health checks and screening can lead to early identification and therefore earlier treatment of conditions.

---

[*] The body's reduced responsiveness to insulin, potentially leading to higher than normal blood sugar levels.

[†] Measured by body mass index (BMI) and/or central obesity. BMI is calculated by dividing a person's body mass by the square of their body height. A large waistline ($\geq$ 40 in/102 cm for men and $\geq$ 35 in/89 cm for women) is a measure of central obesity. This body type is also known as "apple-shaped," as opposed to "pear-shaped," in which fat is deposited on the hips and buttocks. Apple-shaped people are known to be more at risk for cardiometabolic disease than pear-shaped people. A CDC resource on weight is included in **Useful web resources**.

Aging with spastic quadriplegia

As we grow older, our beauty fades physically,
but our inner beauty shines even more brightly.
Unknown

Adults with spastic quadriplegia have had their CP since childhood, but they are also susceptible to the same challenges of aging as their nondisabled peers. For the individual with spastic quadriplegia, it is almost as if, on entering adulthood, two roads converge: the challenges of growing up with their condition meet the challenges of typical aging. Both sets of challenges must be managed in combination. The problems of aging are likely to occur at a younger age and with more severity in adults with CP than in those without the condition.[256] A recent systematic review and meta-analysis of 69 studies from 18 countries found that the prevalence of several chronic physical and mental health conditions was higher among adults with CP than those without CP.[257] However, much can be done to prevent or minimize many of the secondary conditions that can arise.

As in most areas of medicine, the management and treatment of spastic quadriplegia in childhood and adolescence has improved in recent decades. This influences how today's children and adolescents will fare as tomorrow's adults. For example, as we saw in Chapter 2, the risk of hip displacement in spastic quadriplegia is very high; therefore, good hip surveillance programs are an important addition. The general public's awareness of many health issues has also improved.

It is important to note that prevalence rates vary between countries. Using data from the US, Peterson and colleagues reported that the age-adjusted prevalence of chronic conditions is higher in adults with CP (all GMFCS levels) compared to adults without CP[258] (see Figure 9.3.1). The three highest conditions reported among adults with CP were joint pain, arthritis, and hypertension (high blood pressure).

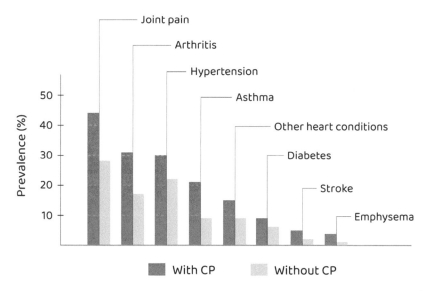

Figure 9.3.1 Age-adjusted prevalence of chronic conditions in adults with and without CP. Data from Peterson and colleagues.[258] **Age-adjusted** refers to a data standardization method to account for differences in ages allowing for more accurate comparison. **Emphysema** is a condition in which the air sacs of the lungs are damaged and enlarged, causing breathlessness.

Some studies have specifically looked at the prevalence of chronic conditions among adults with CP GMFCS levels IV and V. See Tables 9.3.1 and 9.3.2, with data by gender presented in the latter.

Data from a systematic review and meta-analysis of chronic condition prevalence in adults with CP GMFCS levels IV and V is shown in Table 9.3.1.[257]

Table 9.3.1 Prevalence of chronic conditions in adults with CP GMFCS levels IV and V

	PREVALENCE (%)
Constipation	58[259]
Depression	37[259]
Pressure ulcers	28[259]
Epilepsy	26[259]
Underweight	23[257]
Hypercholesterolemia (high cholesterol)	21[257]
Hypertension (high blood pressure)	15[257]
Obesity	14[257]
Anxiety	12[259]

Table 9.3.1 shows that the prevalence of almost all the chronic conditions reported was high in adults with CP GMFCS levels IV and V. Of particular note is the high prevalence of constipation, depression, and pressure ulcers.

A UK study of depression and anxiety found:[260]

- Sixteen percent of adults with CP without intellectual disability and 12 percent with CP with intellectual disability experienced anxiety.
- Twenty percent of adults with CP without intellectual disability and 14 percent of adults with CP with intellectual disability experienced depression.

Many adults with CP GMFCS levels IV and V have an intellectual disability. This study found that those with an intellectual disability are not more likely to develop anxiety or depression compared with adults without CP.[260]

A study by Cremer and colleagues of US adults with CP GMFCS levels IV and V (demographic details in Table 9.3.2) reported chronic condition prevalence by gender as shown in Figure 9.3.2.[261]

Table 9.3.2 Demographics of adults in the Cremer study

	WOMEN	MEN
Number of participants	97	77
Average age (years)	50	50
Body mass index (BMI) kg/m²	27	24
% obese (BMI>30)	30	13
% smokers	9	7

Data from Cremer and colleagues.[261]

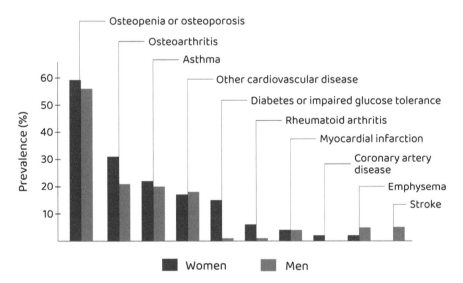

Figure 9.3.2 Prevalence (percent) of chronic conditions in adults with CP GMFCS levels IV and V, by gender. Data from Cremer and colleagues.[261] **Impaired glucose tolerance** refers to a prediabetes condition where blood sugars are higher than normal but not high enough for a diabetes diagnosis. **Rheumatoid arthritis** is an autoimmune condition characterized by inflammation of the joints, causing pain, swelling, and stiffness. **Myocardial infarction** is also known as heart attack.

Figure 9.3.2 shows that, in general, adult women with CP experience a higher burden of chronic conditions than adult men with CP.

"Multimorbidity" is defined as the presence of two or more chronic conditions.[257] The prevalence of multimorbidity was significantly higher among obese than nonobese adults with CP GMFCS levels IV and V (79 percent versus 64 percent).[261]

Collectively this data shows that:

- In addition to their condition which they have had since childhood, adults with CP GMFCS levels IV and V suffer from many further chronic conditions that develop with aging.
- The age-adjusted prevalence of chronic conditions in US adults with CP was higher than in adults without CP.
- The prevalence of most chronic conditions was higher in adult women with CP GMFCS levels IV and V than in men.
- The percentage of adult women with CP who were obese was higher than men. Multimorbidity was found to be high, and it was higher in those who are obese than in those who are not obese.

In summary, in addition to the high burden of their childhood onset condition, adults with spastic quadriplegia GMFCS levels IV and V have a high burden of secondary conditions.

Management and treatment of spastic quadriplegia in adulthood

Grow old with me
The best is yet to be
John Lennon

The general consensus in the literature is that services for adults with CP are extremely limited. Multidisciplinary care teams in place for children and adolescents with CP largely do not exist for adults at a time when their needs are becoming ever more complex. This disparity has been observed in many countries, including Norway,[262] the Netherlands,[263] the US,[249] Ireland,[264] Germany,[265] and Canada.[266] Scandinavian countries are known for their well-developed social health systems, yet other than Sweden,[267] they too experience this fall-off in services. It is very unfortunate that care for people with CP becomes fragmented just as they enter adulthood.

In their 2009 report following a workshop to define the challenges of treating and preventing secondary complications in adults with CP, Tosi and colleagues noted that pediatric facilities are starting to extend their mandate to include adults. They cited Gillette's model of lifetime care.* Gillette provides lifelong specialty care to adolescents and adults who have conditions that began in childhood. This specialization means that even though it is a lifetime care provider, it does not treat lifelong conditions that develop after early childhood.[252]

One very positive development is that a clinical practice guideline for CP in adulthood is being developed. Once published, the guideline will provide a checklist for primary care providers (PCPs), also termed "general practitioners" (GPs), and for adults with CP themselves for managing their health care. Adults with CP and/or their caregivers are encouraged to get and read this guideline and to take it to appointments. (It will be available online through the Cerebral Palsy Foundation.)

Many health care providers often blame a CP diagnosis for just about all of the symptoms and problems that develop in adults with CP.[268,269] Rosenbaum noted: "We hear too many stories from adults with cerebral palsy whose abdominal pain, for example, was assumed to be 'part of [your] cerebral palsy,' when in fact they had treatable Crohn's or gall bladder disease."[269] It is important to ensure that the cause of a health problem is not wrongly attributed to CP when there may be another cause.

Sometimes, changes with aging versus new neurological changes are difficult to separate, especially in adults with CP older than 40 years, but it is important to determine the cause.[270] New neurological changes might include a decreased level of alertness or cognitive functioning, decreased ability to communicate, weakness, or numbness, including paresthesia (pins-and-needles sensation). For example, cervical myelopathy should be considered with new neurological changes. Cervical myelopathy refers to the symptoms related to spinal cord compression (myelopathy) in the neck (cervical) region. Symptoms may include weakness, numbness, loss of fine motor skills, and bladder issues. In addition, dual

---

* The Gillette adult clinic is a lifelong outpatient clinic for those age 16 and older who have conditions that began in childhood. It includes access to an inpatient unit for adults age 18 to 40. Specialists may provide care to adults whom they previously treated as children.

diagnoses (e.g., multiple sclerosis* or even genetic conditions) should also be considered with functional decline.[270]

Much of the philosophy for managing spastic quadriplegia GMFCS levels IV and V in childhood and adolescence, introduced in section 2.3 and detailed in Chapters 3 to 6, remains very relevant for adults. Additions are health screenings and the prevention and management of secondary conditions.

All adults—those with and without disabilities—should attend regular health screenings (e.g., for cancers) and have a regular health check with their primary care provider. Research has found that many adults with CP do not receive adequate screenings and health checks.[252,271,272]

Addressing medical caregivers, Murphy succinctly summarized the situation: "It should be a humbling revelation to all caregivers that this population of adults is almost certainly under-studied, under-screened, and under-diagnosed."[268] (Note that "underdiagnosis" refers to other conditions, not their CP.)

Levi and his siblings turned 15 this summer. This is a bittersweet time for us, and another point in life where grieving the child that might have been is sure to arise. Levi's brother and sister will be getting their driver's permits and likely getting their first jobs. Pretty soon they will apply to colleges and eventually move out on their own and start families. Levi will not do any of those things, though he will make his own important milestones I am sure! Planning for Levi looks different than planning for our other children. We feel strongly that Levi should live with us for as long as we can care for him. My husband and I started strength training and prioritizing fitness about 10 years ago knowing that we will be lifting and caring for Levi for the remainder of our lives. Another important aspect of planning for Levi is ensuring there is money set aside to care for him if we pass away before he does. We are blessed to have a large, close-knit family who we know will care for Levi,

---

* A chronic autoimmune disease of the central nervous system where the immune system mistakenly attacks the myelin, the protective covering of axons, leading to interruption in the transmission of nerve impulses. See Figure 1.2.2.

but we hope to ensure Levi is well taken care of through intentional estate planning well in advance.

As Levi (and we) get older, we will simply do all we can each and every day to ensure his health and happiness for as long as we can. If at the end of the day, Levi feels he is loved and gives us his charming smile before a night of refusing to sleep, we know we did the best we could for him!

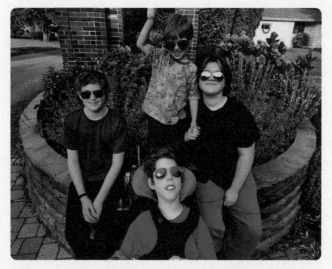

Cam, Levi, Ana, now age 15, with cousin, Finn.

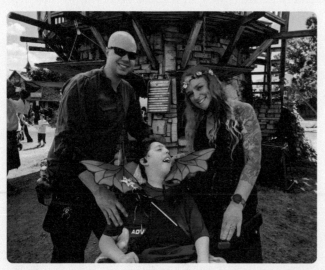

David, Levi, and Kate.

Key points Chapter 9

- CP is diagnosed in childhood and is a lifelong condition. The severity of problems affects life expectancy. However, over the past three decades, data from California has shown that there have been significant improvements in the survival of children with CP and severe disability.
- Many, but not all, individuals with spastic quadriplegia will likely need supported living arrangements and support with decision-making.
- As a person with spastic quadriplegia reaches adulthood and skeletal growth has ceased, a certain stabilization of the musculoskeletal aspects of the condition occurs. The rate of change of the condition is slower in adulthood, assuming the adult remains physically active. Individuals with spastic quadriplegia may, however, develop secondary conditions in adulthood. Some are consistent with typical aging; some may be unique. Each may influence body systems in more complex ways because of the interactions with CP itself.
- Examples of the decline that may occur with typical aging include sarcopenia, joint pain, osteoarthritis, osteoporosis, falls, and low-trauma fractures. Many conditions become more prevalent as people age, including cardiovascular disease, cancer, respiratory disease, and diabetes. These conditions are termed "noncommunicable diseases."
- Adults with spastic quadriplegia have had their condition since childhood, but they are also susceptible to the same challenges of typical aging. For the person with spastic quadriplegia, it is almost as if, on entering adulthood, two roads converge: the challenges of growing up with the condition meet the challenges of typical aging. The two sets of challenges must be managed in combination. The problems of aging may occur at a younger age and with more severity in adults with CP than in those without the condition.
- The prevalence of several chronic physical and mental health conditions was found to be higher among adults with CP than those without CP. However, much can be done to prevent or minimize many of the secondary conditions that can arise.

Chapter 10

Living with spastic quadriplegia

> What lies behind us and what lies before us
> are tiny matters compared to what lies within us.
> **Oliver Wendell Holmes**

In this chapter, people share stories of living with spastic quadriplegia.

Jarett, father of five-year old Julia,
from Minnesota, US

It was November of 2018. In the span of a week, my wife, Erin, was diagnosed with a deadly brain cancer (glioblastoma), my father had a significant stroke, and our younger daughter was diagnosed with microcephaly (and later cerebral palsy). These were such significant events and moments for our entire family, and each one needed its own attention to detail and care, and each demanded such emotional and general processing of the immense ripple effects on our existing life plans, thoughts, and dreams. Everything changed about what we thought the next week, month, and year would and could hold for us.

We received the diagnosis for Julia in a coldly worded letter, clearly stating, "Julia has cerebral palsy." This communication approach was much different from our in-person discussion we had had with the doctors about what might be going on. We had been tracking Julia's progress because we had concerns. She was small, just like her two-and-a-half-year-old sister had been at the same age, but Julia's head size was tracking the very bottom of growth chart, she was not making physical gains like her older sister did, and she was not hitting the typical milestones. We could also see a difference in the way she was progressing compared to her peers at daycare.

After receiving the letter, my wife and I wanted to know the "why": Why does our daughter have cerebral palsy? How did this happen? We embarked on some genetic testing for answers, but it took us nowhere.

Erin was experiencing major "mom guilt," as she felt like she had done something wrong, and what was happening to Julia was her fault in some way. Making it extra difficult was she was processing these feelings alongside her own terminal brain cancer diagnosis. I reminded her of all the times she did everything she could, how she did things right, how she took care of herself and Julia during her pregnancy, how much she loved and cared about Julia—and that none of this was anyone's fault and we needed to change our mindset immediately about Julia no matter what. We needed to acknowledge that Julia is ours, and we know we love her, and will always love her and do our best for her no matter what. There was only one direction to take, and that was forward. That's just the way it was going to be. We agreed that was the case.

Ultimately, after Julia had several CTs and MRIs, and we connected with an amazing medical team at Gillette and the University of Minnesota, it was determined that she has polymicrogyria (a condition where there are too many folds in the brain, and they are unusually small). The cause was an infection from a common virus (CMV) when Julia was in utero, one that Erin had no immunity against. This infection happened at a critical time in Julia's development and changed the way her brain developed. All of that is the root cause of Julia's cerebral palsy.

While that information helped us understand Julia's overall case, it didn't change the fact that we needed to create a plan to deal with Julia the person, our beautiful daughter, and how she experiences the world. We already knew we needed to deal with the symptoms. We already knew she'd need regular speech therapy, physical therapy, occupational therapy, PM&R appointments—and whatever else to keep the doors open for her development. We already knew our lives were forever changed and we'd need to adapt to be the best advocates we could be for Julia.

Julia's diagnosis would prove to be very important for how Erin navigated her four-and-a-half-year journey with brain cancer (much longer than the typical glioblastoma prognosis of 12 months). Being there for Julia was such a motivating factor for Erin. At top of mind—beyond her own cancer treatments, radiation appointments, surgeries, and recoveries—were our girls, especially the things we needed to do for them. For Julia, she would regularly look for used medical equipment, stay on top of therapy appointment scheduling, work on feeding, think of questions we needed to ask, think about Julia's future and what she needed—and just physically give her presence, time, and attention. Julia was not a distraction from Erin's diagnosis; she was a mission, a reason to live. Julia is nonverbal, but she would respond to her mom's love in such expressive ways. With her smile. With her laugh. With her body language. With her whole being.

What our family learned through it all is that we have a lot to learn. We need to remain open and honest. We need to listen to Julia in the form of how she responds to treatments and is developing. We need to be motivated by her attitude, her tenacity, and her infectious smile. We also learned that while there is so much *to* do, there is only so much a person *can* do. Julia's diagnosis and Erin's diagnosis taught us to look forward. To do the things we can. To control the things we can control and, hopefully, realize our own boundaries and the things that are out of our control. We learned we need to be fierce and fair advocates for Julia and kids like her—making sure they are not just surviving but are being given opportunities to thrive on their terms.

Today, Julia is loving kindergarten in her wheelchair, in her gait trainer, with her speech device, and with her friends. She is so happy to be there. It's a milestone that Erin desperately wanted to see and experience here on Earth. It's something I know Julia's infectious smile and laugh—making all those other kids smile and laugh—would warm her heart. It warms my heart, and I can't wait to see what's next for Julia.

John, father of 17-year-old David, from Luxembourg

One day when we were waiting at the airport for the wheelchair assistance to board our plane, an elderly lady looked at our son, David, who has cerebral palsy and was about 12 at the time, then turned to us and asked if we had any other children. "No," we answered. "I'm so sorry for you," she said. Her embarrassed husband told her to show more consideration. But the old lady only said what many people think when they see the family of a child with spastic quadriplegia.

Fifteen percent of the world's population has some form of disability, but few have to deal with a challenge as complex and all-consuming as spastic quadriplegia. After an intensive start, parenting for most people gets easier as their children grow in ability and autonomy. But for those who have a child with spastic quadriplegia, that period of intensive parenting never ends. A person of any age who cannot eat, drink, dress, shower, use the toilet, or perform other basic functions independently requires the same level of assistance as an infant, even if in terms of intellect and spirit they are far more capable. They can also be more demanding.

Our own story began as most cases of cerebral palsy do: with a period in the neonatal intensive care unit. We do not know what caused the problem, but we do know that the placenta had calcified and our son David had to be brought into the world by cesarean section a month earlier than planned. We have lingering doubts about the way he was handled in the hours following the birth and whether this caused or exacerbated the brain injury, but it's too late to determine this now.

When David was about six months old, his pediatrician voiced concern about our son's development and sent us to a neurologist, who said that he was just tense. We visited a physiotherapist who specialized in working with children and who told us that, on the contrary, there was something not at all right about his development. At the time, it was the middle of the summer and difficult to get a doctor's appointment. So we started doing our own research and came to the conclusion that David has cerebral palsy. This initial experience taught us to be confident about educating ourselves in our son's condition and to value the opinions of all the different professionals working with our son.

Luxembourg is a small country with a population of a bit more than half a million when our son was born. On average, only two babies with spastic quadriplegia were born there each year, so it's not surprising that there was no network of parents for us to turn to (we have since remedied that). We started to look to other countries for information (I have Irish and British nationality, and my wife is Portuguese). That is how I became involved in the International Cerebral Palsy Society.

We started visiting the specialized cerebral palsy center in Lisbon. Compared with Luxembourg, one of the richest countries in the world with very generous social security, Portugal is a poor cousin. The public health system is underfunded and people often have to fundraise to buy mobility equipment. Yet the concentration of professionals from different disciplines working together in the CP center, together with the number of children they treat, gives them a level of expertise far higher than we found in Luxembourg. Money can certainly help, but it isn't the only answer to getting the best treatment and advice for your child with spastic quadriplegia.

The old lady at the airport did not know David. If she had, instead of seeing a helpless boy in a wheelchair, she would have recognized a determined, ambitious, positive-minded youngster who will not let any obstacle get in his way. David does not feel sorry for himself because he uses a wheelchair (he is GMFCS level IV). That is just his baseline in life, and from there he sees every new piece of mobility equipment, assistive technology device, or inclusive activity as another opportunity to live life to the fullest.

In *A Midsummer Night's Dream*, Shakespeare tells the story of a "changeling boy." According to folklore, children with disabilities—changelings—are switched by fairies for able-bodied children. Yet rather than suffer abuse, which was the sad fate of many changelings, the boy in Shakespeare's play is desired and lavished with love. That's been our experience with our David.

Parents of a child with any disability, especially spastic quadriplegia, will go through a grieving process for the child they will not have. Looking after a child with a disability is hard work, and many parents find it difficult to cope. But with all the challenges, we have also gained fortitude, resilience, a different perspective on the world, and a deeper understanding of parental love. That is a gift.

Kristen, mother of 20-year-old Avery, from Minnesota, US

Avery was born at 29 weeks due to placenta abruption,* and she spent six weeks in the NICU. During her time there, a head ultrasound was performed that revealed cystic periventricular leukomalacia (PVL),† which her doctors attributed to oxygen deprivation before delivery. She was seen by specialists in ophthalmology, developmental pediatrics, and physical medicine and rehabilitation both while in the NICU and after leaving the hospital.

After having missed many milestones and showing irregularities in her muscle tone, Avery was diagnosed with spastic quadriplegia when she was 10 months old. Receiving the diagnosis allowed us to create a solid plan for moving forward. In addition to the specialists she was already seeing, other specialists and therapists were added to establish her baseline and follow her progress.

Over the years, Avery has had 32 surgeries and numerous tests and procedures, largely related to her CP. We have entered into each surgery with confidence in her medical team and in our knowledge and understanding of her situation at that point in time. We've sought out second opinions when necessary to provide us with reassurance in our plan.

The many appointments can be overwhelming and, at times, annoying, but keep in mind that these professionals want to help your child reach their full potential. Their recommendations should be backed by science and research, which you can easily confirm by doing a little research of your own. The exercises they recommend may be difficult for your child to do, and there may be tears, but the end goal is for their benefit. Lean on someone you trust and feel comfortable with (e.g., your child's physiatrist) for help in prioritizing the recommendations of the various specialists, especially if you are feeling overwhelmed. Spending time with family and friends, having fun, and relaxing are all important too.

---

* "Placenta abruption" means the placenta detaches from the uterus before the infant is born, with potentially life-threatening risks for both the mother and infant. It requires immediate medical attention.

† Formation of cysts in the white matter around the ventricles in the brain.

Finding balance is the key to physical, social, and emotional well-being for both you and your child.

Avery was provided with special education services from preschool through high school graduation, and she is now in transitional programming. While in school, she spent much of her day receiving individualized instruction in the special ed classroom and was mainstreamed when appropriate. She was blessed to have wonderful teachers, therapists, support staff, and nursing care all along the way. Together, we were a unified team with Avery's best interests at heart. Everyone had a voice and was treated with respect, even if we didn't always agree.

With contributions from various funding sources, Avery is fortunate to have use of equipment that helps her more fully participate in all aspects of life. She has been introduced to adaptive sports through Gillette's therapeutic recreation program, such as waterskiing, downhill skiing, and 5K running races. She has also participated in other adaptive activities including baseball, gymnastics, swimming, and horseback riding. Avery was part of the 2016 Mall of America Back to School Look Book. The book featured a group of children and teens wearing the latest fall attire.

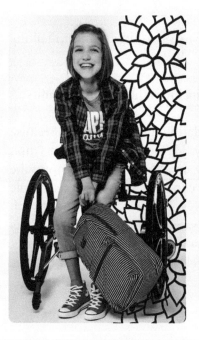
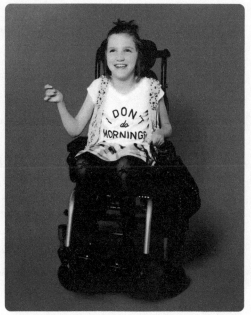

There are so many opportunities for individuals like Avery to live a full and active life.

A diagnosis of CP may feel heavy at times, but your mindset will make all the difference. It's important to be informed about all things CP, and set your focus on what is, instead of what may be in the future.

As challenging as our family life can be, it is also deeply rewarding. Through Avery, we have seen the best humanity has to offer, and we have been blessed in unimaginable and immeasurable ways. When we came to realize that we had been given the incredible opportunity to be Avery's arms and legs and hands and feet, it changed everything. We don't have to take care of her; we get to take care of her, and we get to help her live her best life.

Keoni, age 21, from Australia

Keoni's cerebral palsy doesn't allow him to write his own story, but he can tell it. His family recorded him telling it over a few sessions. These are his own words and thoughts.

I have cerebral palsy. Writing is hard for me, but I can speak to tell my story.

I've discovered things that help me. This includes the ocean and jiujitsu.*

I've been surfing since I was three. My dad taught me to surf. Because of him I grew up in the surf community. He pushed me onto my first wave. Surfing is a way of life, and as they say, "Only a surfer knows the feeling." But surfing with cerebral palsy can be hard. It's not as simple as grabbing a board and hitting the waves. I have a wider board with handles. I use a flotation vest to keep me safe. Surf brands have wetsuits with flotation and flotation vests. I need someone to help me paddle out and catch waves. I also have a beach wheelchair to get me on and off the

---

* A Japanese martial art.

beach. I wasn't always confident to go out in bigger surf; it took a lot of practice and training.

During physio sessions, I learned to swim, practiced paddling my board in the pool, and learned to hold my breath underwater.

What makes surfing so great is the community. Whether I'm with family, friends, or making new friends in the water, it is the best.

I love all sports. I love skiing and have been lucky enough to go to Whistler.*

I started jiujitsu four years ago. I've been hooked ever since, and I'm committed to mastering jiujitsu. I want to compete one day. Jiujitsu helps me exercise and makes me feel good. I don't like missing training. I have my purple belt. Getting it was one of the best days of my life. I've got great coaches who adapt the moves for me. Like surfing, jiujitsu has an incredible community. It's not all easy. This year I changed gyms. I have made great friends.

Finishing high school last year was good and bad. Figuring out what I want to do for a job has been hard. I don't know what I want to do. Throughout school I had a job at a café. It was fun. For now, I'm focused on physio, gym sessions, and jiujitsu classes. I also do a program called Bright Inclusions twice a week and do classes on art, photography, and mindfulness.

I currently rely on a modified car with a ramp for my electric wheelchair, a manual wheelchair for travel, a walker for getting around the house, and a modified bathroom/shower. I wear Nike FlyEase shoes. Before these shoes, it was hard to find shoes that fit my AFOs and they were so hard to put on. Now, I have lots of shoes and a pretty cool shoe collection.

---

* A ski resort in British Columbia, Canada.

I've had nine surgeries including on my knees and back, and I have a shunt.* I don't like hospitals. Hospitals can be hard, not just for me, but for my family. I try to stay positive, but it is hard. I have tough days where my thoughts feel jumbled, and I can't get the right words out.

My whole life I have done physio, OT, and speech therapy. I've tried most things, but I find routine is what helps me the most.

Over the past couple of years, advocating for inclusion has become important to me. I want to help more people. We need a world where everyone who has a disability feels seen and valued.

Kristi, mother of 20-year-old Joe, from Minnesota, US

I had a typical pregnancy with my son, Joe, although I did notice he didn't move around nearly as much as his older sister, Eleanor, had. I had an ultrasound during my pregnancy and that looked good.

Joe was born a week past his due date weighing 6 lb 8 oz. It was a hectic, quick birth with the nurse-midwife and nurses saying that he needed to come out right away because neither his heart rate nor mine was doing well. I was getting oxygen while I was pushing, and I was able to deliver him quickly. Joe initially looked well and his Apgar scores were good. I do remember someone mentioned a "true knot" issue.

I was not aware of how serious the labor and delivery were until one of the nurses came to check on us later. She said, "He looks great. Sometimes the outcome is not good with a true knot issue." I had heard of knots in the umbilical cord before but never a true knot. I started researching what it meant and learned that a true knot is so tight that it can block oxygen and nutrients from reaching the fetus during pregnancy and delivery.

---

* A surgically implanted device that takes excess cerebrospinal fluid from the brain to another part of the body, typically the abdomen.

Joe's first 24-plus hours after delivery were rough. He had difficulty latching on my breast to feed. We also tried a bottle, but he could not do that either. He was very unhappy and cried most of the time and seemed "jittery." Luckily, that same nurse came in later that afternoon and said she was going to try a swing for him to help settle him. The swinging motion didn't help either, so they decided to call the on-call doctor that night as poor Joe had not slept more than a minute here and there since delivery.

They used some drugs to help calm and relax him, and over the next few days, they ran a lot of tests—an EEG, lumbar puncture-spinal tap,* blood tests, and more. Nothing was conclusive on most of his tests: some of his numbers were high, and the EEG showed nothing definite. Finally, after 10 days in the NICU, he was able to join us at home since he was able to nurse better.

No one would officially give me a cerebral palsy diagnosis—they all kept saying, "Let's wait until he is one or older." But when he was not meeting his fine and gross motor skills goals, he was referred to a physiatrist—a doctor of physical medicine and rehab—who officially diagnosed Joe as having spastic quadriplegia cerebral palsy, meaning all four limbs are involved. This started Joe on a journey of appointments for physical therapy, occupational therapy, and speech therapy.

Joe had a very difficult first couple of years as he rarely slept. His naps and nighttime sleep consisted of just a few minutes at a time. When he turned three, he suddenly started sleeping at night, which gave him some much needed rest, but he still would not nap.

As the years went on, we had great support from his various doctors and therapists, as well as the school system. His school therapists encouraged me to seek additional financial help for Joe from from the county and state, and his first few social workers from the county provided advice on things like home modifications needed, getting an adaptive van, and more. I had no idea that we would also need state medical assistance in addition to our primary health insurance for all Joe's expenses.

---

* A lumbar puncture, also known as a spinal tap, is a medical procedure in which a needle is inserted into the spinal canal to collect cerebrospinal fluid.

Joe now has lots of medical equipment that increase his independence—a manual wheelchair, power wheelchair, iPad with a communication app, shower chair, ceiling lift, safety bed, and adaptive bike.

Joe will turn 21 this June and has one more year in his school's transition program, which helps him and his fellow students with writing résumés, filling out job applications, meal planning, grocery shopping, finding housing, managing money, and much more to help them in their daily lives.

The past 21 years have been hard and stressful, but also wonderful, exciting, and amazing to see how far Joe has come. He participates in adaptive sports such as hippotherapy, downhill adaptive skiing on a bi-ski, adaptive waterskiing, bike riding, and many other activities. It's great to be living in Minnesota as the state has recently increased the transition program age to 22 and offers adaptive sports for boys and girls (grades 7 through 12) with physical or cognitive impairments.

Joe is a very social and busy guy; he was elected the Fire and Ice King during his senior year in high school, and he was an honorary member of the boys' state basketball team in his junior and senior years. He runs an annual lemonade stand fundraiser every summer to raise money for an adaptive bike fund. He loves being a part of the community and was recently awarded Richfield's Citizen of the Year for his contributions.

My advice to other families is to always speak up and advocate for your child whether they are a baby or an adult. It's not an easy journey, but always ask questions and reach out to others for advice and help. It's wonderful to have so many great groups you can find online through social media and other organizations that can help answer your questions. In turn, you can also give advice and feedback to others.

Danielle, an adult from Minnesota, US

I celebrated my 40th birthday in December 2023. With every birthday I celebrate, I look back and realize what an amazing thing it is I am alive. In 1983, when I was born at 29 weeks gestation, there were not all the technologies and medications to help preemies survive and thrive that we have today. In addition, I had severe bleeding on the left side of my brain. Despite that, and despite weighing only 2 lb 12 oz, I was breathing room air within 24 hours. Doctors warned my mom I would have deficits, but they didn't know what or how severe they would be. I was in the NICU until the end of February 1984, and then I came home.

When I was nine months old, I had my first physical therapy and occupational therapy evaluations. It was then I was diagnosed with spastic quadriplegic cerebral palsy. That was the earliest age they would do the evaluations, but Mom has told me she knew well before then because of the doctors' warning and by the way I was moving my body and holding my hands. I don't remember much about the interventions that took place when I was really young, but one thing I do vividly remember was having to do side sitting in physical therapy, which was intended to help strengthen my head and trunk control. I absolutely despised doing it! To this day, when I see someone side sitting, it makes me cringe.

I also remember that when I got a little bit older, I couldn't get enough of using a standing frame. It was only something I did at school, and I never wanted to get out of it. It was something I did every day during class. It was amazing to see the world from such a different perspective. Another stand-out memory is from occupational therapy when they allowed me to play with shaving cream to help me get used to different textures. From that point on, I came home asking Mom to put shaving cream on the lap tray on my wheelchair. She would always do it, but she was never excited about cleaning it up!

I got my first power chair when I was six years old. That was a big time in my life because, up until then, I was either carried or pushed everywhere in a manual chair. Once I had my power chair, I could move by myself. It felt sort of like I had my own version of legs. The brand was Hot Wheels, which I think is kind of funny now. It was my own Hot Wheels car that could go forward, back, left, and right when I put my left index finger on the joystick. I remember feeling a sense of freedom I had never felt before. I could now play outside with my siblings without Mom having to be around to push me in my chair, or watch the games my peers were playing during recess without having to tell someone where I wanted to be taken on the playground. Wherever I was, I could navigate independently if I was in my chair.

In school, I was always mainstreamed. I had a few close friends in elementary school, and all of them had disabilities. I didn't really have the opportunity to make a lot of friends with typical kids because the playground, where kids typically socialize the most at school, was completely inaccessible to me. I remember driving my wheelchair to the same spot every day at recess. There, I would sit and spin circles because it was my way of being able to go down a slide or fly high on a swing. None of the typical kids interacted with me because they all had their own friends, and I think most of them were scared of my wheelchair. That started to change in third grade. The teacher I had that year has a son with autism, and she was not afraid to constantly remind the class that I was no different than they were just because my arms and legs didn't work like theirs. One day during our regular storytime after lunch, I fell asleep. When I woke up, my nose was running and my educational assistant (EA), who usually helped me with things like wiping my nose, was not back from lunch. My teacher didn't hesitate to go get a Kleenex and wipe my nose. As she was doing this, she pointed out to the class that you can't catch CP. After that, a lot of kids started trying to interact with me more. It still felt like they didn't know what to do when they were with me, though. It still felt like I was scaring them because of my chair.

Middle school was pretty uneventful because by that point I wasn't doing any therapies as I had stopped making progress toward goals in fifth grade. No one, including me, saw any point in continuing when it was clear my motor patterns were already developed. The kids in middle school were more willing to try to interact with me. Maybe it was because some of them had been in school with me before, or maybe it was because they were more mature. Or maybe it was a combination of both. Whatever the reason, I started to build friendships that I felt were genuine and possibly long-lasting. The one thing that stayed the same was I had an EA for the entire day, every day.

In 1999, when I was 15 years old, I got my first intrathecal baclofen (ITB) pump. Like my first power chair, this was a life-changing device. Prior to getting it, I had so much spasticity in my legs I could snap foot plates on my wheelchairs in half because I was pushing so hard on them all the time. (We had to reinforce them with a metal bar to prevent that from happening.) ITB pumps were relatively new when I got mine, so my catheter that puts the medication into my spinal fluid was placed very low in my lumbar region. That meant that I saw more spasticity reduction in my legs than in my arms. Still, getting the pump was and continues to be one of the best medical decisions my mom and I ever made. I am not breaking foot plates anymore, and Mom doesn't feel like she is breaking my legs when she is trying to do anything with them.

High school was interesting. I had been on an individualized education plan (IEP) since kindergarten. This told all my teachers what accommodations I needed to succeed in school. For example, I needed worksheets printed out in a larger font so I could see them, and I needed enlarged textbooks. But things didn't always go smoothly. I had a science teacher threaten to send me to detention for not paying attention. I *was* paying attention, but I use only one eye at a time because of the brain damage, and he didn't happen to be looking at the one I was using. We had to bring my eye doctor into an IEP meeting and have him add an addendum saying I used only one at a time. After that situation was resolved, there was prom. Mom and I made my prom outfit: a bright pink skirt and top. We put Velcro on the back of both of them so they were easy to get off. Wearing a traditional dress or skirt would have been impossible because they would have been far too long when I was sitting down, and my arms are too spastic to get in most dress material without it ripping. Prom was another one of those events I wasn't really able to be involved in because the gym was too crowded for me to mingle with people the way I wanted to. But I had fun watching all the people make up silly dance moves, and I enjoyed having a reason to get dressed up. I graduated from high school in May 2004.

I have been in college since 2018. I am doing it online at Southern New Hampshire University. I graduated with my associate degree in December 2023. Currently, I am working on my bachelor's degree in creative writing with an emphasis on fiction so that I can someday write books for children and young adults that demonstrate that, even though we all look and act differently on the outside, we all have the same innate longing for acceptance and understanding from the world around us. I do all my work on my computer using built-in assistive technology. It allows me to interact with my computer using my voice. Without growing up in an era when technology is so prevalent, I wouldn't be able to say I am a college graduate or go back for another degree.

When I am not busy doing schoolwork, I spend time with my nieces and nephew. They know that I do things differently, and they know that I need help with almost everything, unless it involves driving my chair or doing something on my computer. All three of them are very good at adapting the things they play when they are with me so I can be involved. My chair doesn't really faze them because they have all been around it their entire lives. My nephew does get a little irritated when we go places and I'm not able to do things because they are inaccessible. Sometimes he asks, "Why isn't there a way for D to do this?" This happens most when we go to parks or playgrounds where he and his sister can play on the equipment while their mom and I have to sit at a picnic table and watch them because there is nothing I am able to do. I think he is going to grow up and find ways to make the world more accessible for me and other people with similar abilities. He's going to make the change he wants to see!

I've mentioned my mom here often. We are extremely close. Part of that is because she does almost all my caretaking. We have been a team my entire life. I wouldn't be the person I am today and I wouldn't be where I am today without her. She never treated me any different than my siblings when it came to her expectations. If I was being mouthy, she didn't hesitate to pick me up and put me in my room just like she would do with my siblings. I never got any special treatment because of my disability. I feel her lack of special treatment is a big reason why I came to accept my disability as a child, and it's a big part of why I can be such a strong advocate for myself today.

If you have read this far, you may be wondering if I ever have any desire to walk. No, I don't. I have three things, and with those three things I will go anywhere and do anything. I have my brain, my mouth, and six good wheels. I don't need my arms and legs to work like the typical person to change the world. I know writing something like this and having a diverse group of people reading it will change hearts and minds. My hope is that at least one person who reads this will gain a new perspective and plant the seed for someone else who may not know how to interact with someone who has CP or who may be uncomfortable doing so. If that happens for one person, I feel I have done what God put me here to do. I know I'm going to change the world by changing perspectives one reader at a time!

Chapter 11

Further reading and research

Education is not the filling of a pail, but the lighting of a fire.
William Butler Yeats

Further reading

For those who would like further reading on this condition, a list of recommended books, websites, and resources has been collated and will be regularly updated. Access to the list is provided in **Useful web resources.**

Research

Research serves as a cornerstone of evidence-based medicine and drives health care advancement. We discussed the importance of evidence-based medicine (or evidence-based practice) in Chapter 2. It is "the conscientious, explicit, and judicious use of current best evidence in making decisions about the care of individual patients." It combines the best available external clinical evidence from research with the clinical expertise of the professional.[83] Family priorities and preferences are also considered.[84]

Evidence is collected by carrying out scientific studies (research studies), the results of which are published as full-length, peer-reviewed research articles (or papers) in scientific journals. "Peer-reviewed" means that experts with relevant content knowledge have reviewed, challenged, and agreed that the scientific method and study conclusions based on the results are sound.

Scientific studies may also be presented in brief at conferences, and conference proceedings are often published. However, conference proceedings present preliminary results and peer review is minimal. *Therefore, full-length published research articles are the most rigorous and sound evidence.*

The above published research outputs are collectively known as scientific literature or, simply, research.

Research may also be discussed on various social media platforms such as X (formerly Twitter), Facebook, LinkedIn, and Instagram. If you consume information this way, it is always important to go back to the original source (i.e., the full-length research article) to ensure the media's portrayal of the study findings is accurate.

You may have familiarity with searching the scientific literature. If not, search engines such as PubMed (ncbi.nlm.nih.gov/pubmed) and Google Scholar (scholar.google.com) are good places to start. They provide a free abstract (a short summary of the article), which can be very useful. In the past, you generally needed to belong to an academic or medical institution to have access to full-length research articles. Many articles are now available online for free. Google Scholar provides links to many full-length articles, and some community libraries allow you to request full-length articles.

You might have heard the phrase, "Just because someone says it, doesn't mean it's true." This is worth remembering in all aspects of life, but it is also relevant to research. While research articles go through a peer review process, you should still read them with a critical eye. Ask yourself, How confident can I be in the results of this research study? Was the sample size big enough to be representative of the larger population? Did the results support the conclusion?

If you aren't a trained scientist, reviewing the quality of the evidence might be more challenging, but you can still make sure the basic methods make sense and the author's conclusions are supported by the data presented. The information below will help you learn about some research study designs and how study design affects how much confidence you can place in a study's conclusions.

Research study design

There are different research study designs, and each has its value. The quality of the evidence, or level of evidence, is graded based on the study design and how well the methods were executed. Research articles sometimes list (often in the abstract) the level of evidence from I to V, with level I being the highest.

The most common research study designs, listed from highest to lowest level of evidence, are:

- Systematic review
- Randomized controlled trial
- Cohort
- Case control
- Cross-sectional
- Case report and case series

Systematic review: A systematic review summarizes the results of several scientific studies on the same topic. They can be qualitative (descriptive) or quantitative (numerical):

- Qualitative: A summary of common themes and findings across studies but without a statistical analysis.
- Quantitative: A statistical analysis carried out that takes a weighted average of the findings across studies to produce one estimate for the effect of a treatment, for example. The quantitative approach is called a "meta-analysis."

The highest level of evidence is a systematic review of randomized controlled trials (described next), although systematic reviews can also include studies that used other types of study designs. Systematic reviews may be published by individual researchers or groups. The Cochrane collaboration is a worldwide association of researchers, health care professionals, patients, and carers that publishes systematic reviews on various topics.

Randomized controlled trial (RCT): An RCT is a study design aimed at identifying cause and effect. The cause is, for example, the treatment, and the effect is the outcome being measured. Strict control of the study method (the "C" in RCT) helps to ensure the treatment of interest is the only factor that could cause the outcome. A treatment group receives the treatment while a nontreatment group (also known as the control group) does not. The participants are randomly assigned (the "R" in RCT) to one of the groups. The random assignment is one of the key strengths of this study design because it takes care of the "unknown unknowns" that may influence the outcome. The treatment effect is found by comparing the outcomes of the treatment and nontreatment groups. RCTs are considered the highest quality study design but are still uncommon in medical literature.

Cohort: A cohort is a group of people who share a common characteristic (e.g., diagnosis, gender). In a cohort study, outcome is measured two or more times. Researchers identify the characteristic of interest and then measure the outcome, looking for associations between the two. A cohort study is a form of longitudinal study ("longitudinal" means that the same outcome is measured on the same participants two or more times over a period of time). You may come across the terms "prospective" and "retrospective" cohort studies.

- In prospective cohort studies, research questions and methods are defined, and a cohort is followed over time, collecting data.
- In retrospective cohort studies, research questions and methods are defined after data has been collected or already exists (e.g., a person's medical record).

Case control: In case control studies, researchers identify the outcome of interest, which defines the groups (e.g., infants with a specific diagnosis and typically developing infants), and then look backward in time at different factors or exposures that might have caused different outcomes. At the beginning of the study, the outcome is known, but the factors or exposures that might have caused that outcome are unknown. This is the opposite of cohort studies. Because the outcome and factors or exposures data already exist, case control studies are always retrospective.

Cross-sectional: Cross-sectional studies take measurements only once from participants. Researchers look for associations between certain factors and exposures, and outcomes.

Case report and case series: A case report (also referred to as a single-subject case study) is an account of a single patient—usually a unique case—and their medical history, status, and outcomes from a treatment, for example. A case series is a group of case reports on patients who were exposed to a similar treatment. These reports are usually retrospective, and data has already been collected by other means (usually as part of routine medical care).

Getting involved in research

There are many opportunities to become involved in research. Together with medical professionals and researchers, people with lived experience can help drive advancement in health care.

a) As a participant

Researchers working in academic and medical settings are always looking for participants for their studies. You might receive an invitation to participate in such a study via an email, letter in the mail, phone call, social media ad, or other method.

Some studies are very easy and may just involve completing one online survey; others may take more time with various measurements being taken on more than one occasion. Just as you are advised to read published research studies with a critical eye, so should you judge new research study opportunities before agreeing to participate. Participating can take time and effort—the expected time commitment will be communicated in the study recruitment material. There is often a small reimbursement offered for time spent in a study.

It's worth noting that you, as the study participant, may not personally benefit from the research study, but the collective population with the condition will likely benefit.

Clinical trials are research studies conducted to evaluate the safety and effectiveness of new medical treatments, including new medications and devices before they can be approved for widespread use. They are often conducted following a randomized controlled trial research study design.

A potential benefit of participating in clinical trials is gaining early access to new medical treatments. Even if you are assigned to the control group (which usually receives standard care), you may have early access to the new treatment once the data collection phase is complete. In addition, standard care is likely to be current best practice.

You can find information about clinical trials through various sources:

- The National Institutes of Health in the US maintains a comprehensive database, ClinicalTrials.gov, where you can learn about clinical trials around the world. You can search this database by specific medical condition, location, or other pertinent criteria to identify relevant clinical trials that may be currently enrolling participants.
- Major academic medical centers, research institutions, and hospitals often conduct clinical trials and can provide information about their ongoing studies.
- Medical professionals may be aware of ongoing clinical trials in their field and can provide guidance to families who are interested in participating.
- Organizations that support particular conditions are another source of information.

Depending on the nature of the treatment in the clinical trial, you may want to, or be required to, consult with your medical professional to help you consider the risks and benefits of participating.

b) As a co-producer

Family engagement in research (FER) plays a crucial role in fostering collaboration and helping improve study design and outcome. When families become involved in research as collaborators on a study rather than simply as participants, researchers gain valuable insights into the lived experiences and perspectives of families. Families participate at every stage of the research process: concept, design, planning, conduct, and reporting of the study findings. These opportunities are still rare but are becoming more common. As an example, a link to the FER program at Gillette Children's is included in **Useful web resources**.

The family engagement in research movement is largely attributed to the similar and earlier patient and public involvement initiative in the UK. Here are some opportunities:

- **CanChild** and the **Kids Brain Health Network** in Canada currently offer The Family Engagement in Research program, a short online training course through McMaster University Continuing Education, to train family members and researchers (including coordinators and assistants) in collaborating on research.
- Online training modules are available at **Patient-Oriented Research Curriculum in Child Health (PORCCH)**.
- The **Patient-Centered Outcomes Research Institute (PCORI)** and the **Strategy for Patient-Oriented Research (SPOR)** are two other organizations that encourage family engagement.

USEFUL WEB RESOURCES

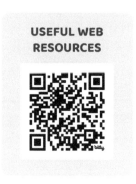

Acknowledgments

It takes a village to raise a child

African proverb

And it takes a village to produce a Healthcare Series. Publication of this series began with an idea, then with five titles, and then more titles. These acknowledgments relate to the entire series.

The formula of deep medical information interspersed with lived experience gives readers an appreciation of the childhood-acquired, often lifelong conditions. We thank the many people who contributed to each title: medical professionals at Gillette Children's who willingly came forward to lead each book; Gillette writers who did the research and writing of each, including Michaela Hingtgen who contributed to this book in the early stages; other Gillette team members who contributed from their different specialties; family authors and vignette writers who shared their personal stories; other families who shared photographs; the Gillette editing team who ensured the content and structure worked for the reader; Olwyn Roche who beautifully illustrated each title; advance readers, both professionals and families, whose feedback was invaluable; and Lina Abdennabi who coordinated Gillette Press operations. Behind every book was also a pit team who converted the finished manuscript into the book you now hold. Ruth Wilson led and looked after copyediting and proofreading. Jazmin Welch created the beautiful design and layout. Audrey McClellan indexed each title.

Smoothly creating each title required great teamwork among our villagers.

Staff at Gillette Children's provided continual support to the project and everyone involved. This included the steering committee, in particular Paula Montgomery, Dr. Micah Niermann, and Barbara Joers.

This Healthcare Series is co-published with Mac Keith Press. From the get-go, the journey with Ann-Marie Halligan and Sally Wilkinson was one of great support and collaboration.

Gillette Children's Healthcare Press

Glossary

Grasp the subject, the words will follow.

Cato the Elder

TERM	DEFINITION
Abnormal/atypical	Deviating from the typical expectation.
Achilles tendon	The cord-like structure that attaches the gastrocnemius and soleus muscles (both calf muscles) to the bone at the heel.
Ankle-foot orthosis (AFO)	A type of orthosis (brace or splint) that controls the ankle and foot. See *orthosis*.
Baclofen	A medication used for tone reduction; can be delivered either orally or by using a pump connected to a catheter to deliver the medication to the intrathecal area (the fluid-filled space surrounding the spinal cord). The latter delivery method is called *intrathecal baclofen* (ITB).
Bilateral CP	A form of cerebral palsy that affects both sides of the body.
Botulinum neurotoxin A (BoNT-A)	A medication used for tone reduction. It is delivered by injection directly into the muscle.
Cardiometabolic	Referring to both heart disease and metabolic disorders (such as diabetes).
Casting	The process of stretching a muscle by applying a plaster of paris or a fiberglass cast; for example, a below-knee cast to stretch the tight gastrocnemius and/or soleus muscles (calf muscles) to hold the muscle in a position of maximum stretch.

Centers for Disease Control and Prevention (CDC)	The national public health institute in the US.
Cerebral	Referring to the cerebrum, the front and upper part of the brain, one of the major areas responsible for the control of movement.
Cobb angle	The angle between the two most tilted vertebrae at the upper and lower ends of a spinal curve.
Contracture	A limitation of the range of motion (ROM) of a joint. It occurs in the muscle-tendon unit (MTU) and/or capsule of the joint, not just the muscle. See *muscle-tendon unit; range of motion.*
Deep brain stimulation (DBS)	A neurosurgical procedure that involves implanting electrodes in specific areas of the brain to reduce dystonia.
Diplegia	A form of cerebral palsy affecting all limbs, but the lower limbs are much more affected than the upper limbs, which frequently show only fine motor impairment.
Drooling	Excess saliva dropping uncontrollably from the mouth.
Dysphagia	Difficulty and/or discomfort in swallowing.
Dystonia	Characterized by involuntary muscle contractions that cause slow repetitive movements or abnormal postures that can sometimes be painful.
Enteral feeding	Also known as tube-feeding, it is liquid nutrition delivered via a feeding tube, a plastic tube, directly into the stomach or small intestine.
Epilepsy	A neurological disorder in which brain activity becomes abnormal, causing seizures or periods of unusual behavior, sensations, and sometimes loss of awareness. See *seizure.*
Episode of care (EOC)	A period of therapy (at the appropriate frequency) followed by a therapy break.

Fine motor function	Refers to the smaller movements in the wrists, hands, fingers, and toes. Examples include picking up objects between the thumb and forefinger, and writing. Also called fine motor skills, hand skills, fine motor coordination, or dexterity.
Gait	A person's manner of walking.
Gastrojejunostomy tube (G-J-tube)	Two tubes in one, surgically inserted with one tube routing to the stomach (G) and the other to the small intestine (J) for delivering nutrition.
Gastrostomy tube (G-tube)	A tube surgically inserted to carry nutrition to the stomach.
Gross motor function	The ability to make large, general movement of the arms, legs, and other large body parts, such as sitting, crawling, standing, running, jumping, swimming, throwing, catching, and kicking. Also called gross motor skills.
Gross Motor Function Classification System (GMFCS)	A five-level classification system that describes the functional mobilities of children and adolescents with cerebral palsy. Level I has the fewest limitations and level V has the most. It provides an indication of the severity of cerebral palsy.
Hemiplegia	A form of cerebral palsy affecting the upper and lower limbs on one side of the body. The upper limb is usually more affected than the lower limb.
Hip displacement (subluxation, dislocation)	The degree to which the head (ball) of the femur (thigh bone) is out of the acetabulum (socket) of the hip bone. With subluxation, the ball is partially out of the socket but is still in contact with it; it is still partially covered by the socket. With dislocation, the ball is completely out of the socket.
Hypotonia/hypertonia	See *muscle tone.*
International Classification of Functioning, Disability and Health (ICF)	A universal framework for considering any health condition. It helps show the impact of a health condition at different levels and how those levels are interconnected.
Intrathecal baclofen (ITB)	Refers to the method of delivering baclofen directly to the cerebrospinal fluid in the intrathecal space.

Jaundice	A yellowing of the skin or whites of the eyes arising from excess of the pigment bilirubin, a yellow pigment formed in the liver by the breakdown of red blood cells and excreted in bile.
Jejunostomy tube (J-tube)	A tube surgically inserted to carry nutrition to the jejunum (a section of the small intestine).
Magnetic resonance imaging (MRI)	A noninvasive imaging technology that produces detailed three-dimensional anatomical images without the use of radiation.
Muscle-tendon unit (MTU)	A combination of the muscle, tendon, and other structures.
Muscle tone	The resting tension in a person's muscles. Tone is considered abnormal when it falls outside the range of normal or typical; either too low (hypotonia) or too high (hypertonia). Abnormal muscle tone occurs in all types of cerebral palsy.
Musculoskeletal	Referring to both the muscles and the skeleton; includes muscles, bones, joints, and their related structures (e.g., ligaments, and tendons). The term *neuromusculoskeletal* includes the nervous system.
Nasogastric tube (NG tube)	A tube inserted through the nose and carries nutrition to the stomach.
Neurology	Specialty dealing with disorders of the nervous system.
Neuromusculoskeletal	Referring to the nervous system, muscles, bones, joints, and their related structures.
Neurosurgery	Specialty that involves surgical management of disorders of the nervous system.
Occupational therapy	A type of therapy based on engaging in everyday activities (occupations) to promote health, well-being, and independence.
Oral feeding	Food and drink taken by mouth.
Orthopedic surgery	Specialty that involves surgical management of disorders affecting the *musculoskeletal* system.

Orthosis	A device designed to hold specific body parts in position to modify their structure and/or function; also called a brace or splint.
Orthotics	The branch of medicine concerned with the design, manufacture, and management of orthoses. See *orthosis*.
Osteoporosis	A medical condition where the bones are weak and brittle, with low density.
Palsy	Paralysis (though paralysis by pure definition is not a feature of cerebral palsy).
Pediatrics	Specialty dealing with children and their conditions.
Percentile	A variable (such as a person's height by age) that divides the distribution of the variable into 100 groups. The 50th percentile is always the median (the midpoint that separates lower and higher values into two groups).
Phenol	A medication used for tone reduction. It is delivered by injection.
Physiatry	See *physical medicine and rehabilitation*.
Physical medicine and rehabilitation (PM&R)	Specialty that aims to enhance and restore functional ability and quality of life among those with physical disabilities. Also termed *physiatry*.
Physical therapy/ physiotherapy	A type of therapy to develop, maintain, and restore a person's maximum movement and functional ability.
Quadriplegia	A form of cerebral palsy affecting all four limbs and the trunk; also known as tetraplegia.
Range of motion (ROM)	A measure of joint flexibility; the range through which a joint moves, measured in degrees. Also called range of movement.
Seizure	Uncontrolled, abnormal electrical activity of the brain that may cause changes in the level of consciousness, behavior, memory, or feelings
Selective dorsal rhizotomy (SDR)	Refers to the selective cutting of abnormal sensory nerve rootlets in the spinal cord to reduce spasticity.

Scoliosis	A three-dimensional rotation and curvature of the spine.
Sialorrhea	Excess saliva.
Spasticity	A condition in which there is an abnormal increase in muscle tone or stiffness of muscle that can interfere with movement and speech, and be associated with discomfort or pain.
Speech and language pathology (SLP)	A type of therapy to support those with speech, language, and communication needs as well as feeding and swallowing difficulties. Also called speech and language therapy.
Tendon	The cord-like structure that attaches the muscle to the bone; for example, the *Achilles tendon* attaches both calf muscles to the bone at the heel.
Tone	See *muscle tone.*
Unilateral CP	A form of cerebral palsy that affects one side of the body.
Ventral dorsal rhizotomy	A neurosurgical procedure that reduces spasticity and dystonia by cutting both the dorsal and ventral nerve rootlets in the spinal cord.
Windswept hips	Abduction and external rotation of one hip, with the opposite hip in adduction and internal rotation. Derives its name from its appearance, as if the person's body had been blown that direction by a strong wind.

References

1. World Health Organization (2001) *International classification of functioning, disability and health (ICF)*. [online] Available at: <https://www.who.int/standards/classifications/international-classification-of-functioning-disability-and-health> [Accessed February 22 2024].

2. Rosenbaum P, Paneth N, Leviton A, et al. (2007) A report: The definition and classification of cerebral palsy April 2006. *Dev Med Child Neurol Suppl*, 109, 8–14.

3. Graham HK, Rosenbaum P, Paneth N, et al. (2016) Cerebral palsy. *Nat Rev Dis Primers*, 2, 1–24.

4. Smithers-Sheedy H, Waight E, Goldsmith S, McIntyre S (2023) Australian Cerebral Palsy Register report, Available at: <https://cpregister.com/wp-content/uploads/2023/01/2023-ACPR-Report.pdf> [Accessed June 24 2024].

5. McIntyre S, Goldsmith S, Webb A, et al. (2022) Global prevalence of cerebral palsy: A systematic analysis. *Dev Med Child Neurol*, 64, 1494–1506.

6. Centers for Disease Control and Prevention (2024a) *Epidemiology glossary*. [online] Available at: <https://www.cdc.gov/reproductive-health/glossary/> [Accessed June 24 2024].

7. Shepherd E, Salam RA, Middleton P, et al. (2017) Antenatal and intrapartum interventions for preventing cerebral palsy: An overview of Cochrane systematic reviews. *Cochrane Database Syst Rev*, 8, 1–78.

8. Rosenbaum P, Rosenbloom L (2012) *Cerebral palsy: From diagnosis to adult life*. London: Mac Keith Press.

9. National Institute of Neurological Disorders and Stroke (2023a) *Cerebral palsy*. [online] Available at: <https://www.ninds.nih.gov/health-information/disorders/cerebral-palsy> [Accessed June 21 2024].

10. Centers for Disease Control and Prevention (2024b) *Risk factors for cerebral palsy*. [online] Available at: <https://www.cdc.gov/cerebral-palsy/risk-factors/> [Accessed June 18 2024].

11. Centers for Disease Control and Prevention (2017) *Single embryo transfer*. [online] Available at: <https://www.cdc.gov/art/patientresources/transfer.html> [Accessed June 24 2024].

12. National Perinatal Epidemiology and Statistics Unit (2021) IVF success rates have improved in the last decade, especially in older women: Report, Australia, UNSW, Available at: <https://www.unsw.edu.au/newsroom/news/2021/09/ivf-success-rates-have-improved-in-the-last-decade--especially-i> [Accessed January 19 2024].

13. Nelson KB (2008) Causative factors in cerebral palsy. *Clin Obstet Gynecol*, 51, 749–62.

14. Novak I, Morgan C, Fahey M, et al. (2020) State of the evidence traffic lights 2019: Systematic review of interventions for preventing and treating children with cerebral palsy. *Curr Neurol Neurosci Rep,* 20, 1–21.

15. Durkin MS, Benedict RE, Christensen D, et al. (2016) Prevalence of cerebral palsy among 8-year-old children in 2010 and preliminary evidence of trends in its relationship to low birthweight. *Paediatr Perinat Epidemiol,* 30, 496–510.

16. McGuire DO, Tian LH, Yeargin-Allsopp M, Dowling NF, Christensen DL (2019) Prevalence of cerebral palsy, intellectual disability, hearing loss, and blindness, national health interview survey, 2009–2016. *Disabil Health J,* 12, 443–451.

17. Khandaker G, Muhit M, Karim T, et al. (2019) Epidemiology of cerebral palsy in Bangladesh: A population-based surveillance study. *Dev Med Child Neurol,* 61, 601–609.

18. Centers for Disease Control and Prevention (2024c) *Down syndrome.* [online] Available at: <https://www.cdc.gov/ncbddd/birthdefects/downsyndrome.html> [Accessed June 21 2024].

19. National Institutes of Health (2024) *Estimates of funding for various research, condition, and disease categories (RCDC).* [online] Available at: <https://report .nih.gov/funding/categorical-spending#/> [Accessed June 21 2024].

20. Mathew JL, Kaur N, Dsouza JM (2022) Therapeutic hypothermia in neonatal hypoxic encephalopathy: A systematic review and meta-analysis. *J Glob Health,* 12, 1–22.

21. Novak I, Morgan C, Adde L, et al. (2017) Early, accurate diagnosis and early intervention in cerebral palsy. *JAMA Pediatr,* 171, 1–11.

22. National Institute of Neurological Disorders and Stroke (2024) *Glossary of neurological terms.* [online] Available at: <https://www.ninds.nih.gov/ health-information/disorders/glossary-neurological-terms> [Accessed June 14 2024].

23. Byrne R, Noritz G, Maitre NL, N.C.H. Early Developmental Group (2017) Implementation of early diagnosis and intervention guidelines for cerebral palsy in a high-risk infant follow-up clinic. *Pediatr Neurol,* 76, 66–71.

24. Maitre NL, Burton VJ, Duncan AF, et al. (2020) Network implementation of guideline for early detection decreases age at cerebral palsy diagnosis. *Pediatrics,* 145, 1–10.

25. Te Velde A, Tantsis E, Novak I, et al. (2021) Age of diagnosis, fidelity and acceptability of an early diagnosis clinic for cerebral palsy: A single site imple-mentation study. *Brain Sci,* 11, 1–14.

26. King AR, Machipisa C, Finlayson F, et al. (2021) Early detection of cerebral palsy in high-risk infants: Translation of evidence into practice in an Australian hospital. *J Paediatr Child Health,* 57, 246–250.

27. King AR, Al Imam MH, McIntyre S, et al. (2022) Early diagnosis of cerebral palsy in low- and middle-income countries. *Brain Sci,* 12, 1–13.

28. Maitre NL, Damiano D, Byrne R (2023) Implementation of early detection and intervention for cerebral palsy in high-risk infant follow-up programs: U.S. And global considerations. *Clin Perinatol,* 50, 269–279.

29. Maitre NL, Byrne R, Duncan A, et al. (2022) "High-risk for cerebral palsy" designation: A clinical consensus statement. *J Pediatr Rehabil Med,* 15, 165–174.

30. Morgan C, Fetters L, Adde L, et al. (2021) Early intervention for children aged 0 to 2 years with or at high risk of cerebral palsy: International clinical practice guideline based on systematic reviews. *JAMA Pediatr*, 175, 846–858.

31. Ismail FY, Fatemi A, Johnston MV (2017) Cerebral plasticity: Windows of opportunity in the developing brain. *Eur J Paediatr Neurol*, 21, 23–48.

32. Cerebral Palsy Alliance (2019) *Why neuroplasticity is the secret ingredient for kids with special needs.* [online] Available at: <https://cerebralpalsy.org.au/news-stories/why-neuroplasticity-is-the-secret-ingredient-for-kids-with-special-needs/> [Accessed June 14 2024].

33. Kohli-Lynch M, Tann CJ, Ellis ME (2019) Early intervention for children at high risk of developmental disability in low- and middle-income countries: A narrative review. *Int J Environ Res Public Health*, 16, 1–9.

34. McNamara L, Morgan C, Novak I (2023) Interventions for motor disorders in high-risk neonates. *Clin Perinatol*, 50, 121–155.

35. Byrne R, Duncan A, Pickar T, et al. (2019) Comparing parent and provider priorities in discussions of early detection and intervention for infants with and at risk of cerebral palsy. *Child Care Health Dev*, 45, 799–807.

36. Centers for Disease Control and Prevention (2024d) *CDC's developmental milestones.* [online] Available at: <https://www.cdc.gov/ncbddd/actearly/milestones/index.html> [Accessed June 21 2024].

37. WHO Multicentre Growth Reference Study Group (2006) WHO motor development study: Windows of achievement for six gross motor development milestones. *Acta Paediatr Suppl*, 450, 86–95.

38. Surveillance of Cerebral Palsy in Europe (2000) A collaboration of cerebral palsy surveys and registers. Surveillance of cerebral palsy in Europe (SCPE). *Dev Med Child Neurol*, 42, 816–24.

39. National Institute of Neurological Disorders and Stroke (2021) *Dystonia [pdf].* [online] Available at: <https://catalog.ninds.nih.gov/sites/default/files/publications/dystonia.pdf> [Accessed January 19 2024].

40. National Institute of Neurological Disorders and Stroke (2023b) *Ataxia and cerebellar or spinocerebellar degeneration.* [online] Available at: <https://www.ninds.nih.gov/health-information/disorders/ataxia-and-cerebellar-or-spinocerebellar-degeneration> [Accessed January 19 2024].

41. Centers for Disease Control and Prevention (2024e) *About cerebral palsy.* [online] Available at: <https://www.cdc.gov/cerebral-palsy/about/> [Accessed June 21 2024].

42. Australian Cerebral Palsy Register (2023) *Personal communication.*

43. Gorter JW, Rosenbaum PL, Hanna SE, et al. (2004) Limb distribution, motor impairment, and functional classification of cerebral palsy. *Dev Med Child Neurol*, 46, 461–7.

44. Himmelmann K, Beckung E, Hagberg G, Uvebrant P (2006) Gross and fine motor function and accompanying impairments in cerebral palsy. *Dev Med Child Neurol*, 48, 417–23.

45. Shevell MI, Dagenais L, Hall N, REPACQ Consortium (2009) The relationship of cerebral palsy subtype and functional motor impairment: A population-based study. *Dev Med Child Neurol*, 51, 872–7.

46. Hidecker MJ, Ho NT, Dodge N, et al. (2012) Inter-relationships of functional status in cerebral palsy: Analyzing gross motor function, manual ability, and communication function classification systems in children. *Dev Med Child Neurol*, 54, 737–42.

47. Aravamuthan BR, Fehlings D, Shetty S, et al. (2021) Variability in cerebral palsy diagnosis. *Pediatrics*, 147, 1–11.

48. Dar H, Stewart K, McIntyre S, Paget S (2023) Multiple motor disorders in cerebral palsy. *Dev Med Child Neurol*, 66, 317–325.

49. Palisano R, Rosenbaum P, Walter S, et al. (1997) Development and reliability of a system to classify gross motor function in children with cerebral palsy. *Dev Med Child Neurol*, 39, 214–23.

50. Palisano RJ, Rosenbaum P, Bartlett D, Livingston MH (2008) Content validity of the expanded and revised Gross Motor Function Classification System. *Dev Med Child Neurol*, 50, 744–50.

51. Alriksson-Schmidt A, Nordmark E, Czuba T, Westbom L (2017) Stability of the Gross Motor Function Classification System in children and adolescents with cerebral palsy: A retrospective cohort registry study. *Dev Med Child Neurol*, 59, 641–646.

52. Huroy M, Behlim T, Andersen J, et al. (2022) Stability of the Gross Motor Function Classification System over time in children with cerebral palsy. *Dev Med Child Neurol*, 64, 1487–1493.

53. McCormick A, Brien M, Plourde J, et al. (2007) Stability of the Gross Motor Function Classification System in adults with cerebral palsy. *Dev Med Child Neurol*, 49, 265–9.

54. Kinsner-Ovaskainen A, Lanzoni M, Martin S, et al. (2017) *Surveillance of cerebral palsy in Europe: Development of the JRC-SCPE central database and public health indicators.* Luxembourg: Publications Office of the European Union.

55. Rosenbaum PL, Walter SD, Hanna SE, et al. (2002) Prognosis for gross motor function in cerebral palsy: Creation of motor development curves. *Jama*, 288, 1357–63.

56. Hanna SE, Bartlett DJ, Rivard LM, Russell DJ (2008) Reference curves for the gross motor function measure: Percentiles for clinical description and tracking over time among children with cerebral palsy. *Phys Ther*, 88, 596–607.

57. Eliasson AC, Krumlinde-Sundholm L, Rösblad B, et al. (2006) The Manual Ability Classification System (MACS) for children with cerebral palsy: Scale development and evidence of validity and reliability. *Dev Med Child Neurol*, 48, 549–54.

58. Eliasson AC, Ullenhag A, Wahlstrom U, Krumlinde-Sundholm L (2017) Mini-MACS: Development of the Manual Ability Classification System for children younger than 4 years of age with signs of cerebral palsy. *Dev Med Child Neurol*, 59, 72–78.

59. Beckung E, Hagberg G (2002) Neuroimpairments, activity limitations, and participation restrictions in children with cerebral palsy. *Dev Med Child Neurol*, 44, 309–16.

60. Elvrum AK, Andersen GL, Himmelmann K, et al. (2016) Bimanual Fine Motor Function (BFMF) classification in children with cerebral palsy: Aspects of construct and content validity. *Phys Occup Ther Pediatr,* 36, 1–16.

61. Elvrum AG, Beckung E, Saether R, et al. (2017) Bimanual capacity of children with cerebral palsy: Intra- and interrater reliability of a revised edition of the Bimanual Fine Motor Function classification. *Phys Occup Ther Pediatr,* 37, 239–251.

62. Hidecker MJ, Paneth N, Rosenbaum PL, et al. (2011) Developing and validating the Communication Function Classification System for individuals with cerebral palsy. *Dev Med Child Neurol,* 53, 704–10.

63. Pennington L, Mjøen T, Da Graça Andrada M, Murray J (2010) Viking Speech Scale [pdf] EU, European Commission, Available at: <https://eu-rd-platform.jrc .ec.europa.eu/sites/default/files/Viking-Speech-Scale-2011-Copyright_EN.pdf> [Accessed June 18 2024].

64. Pennington L, Virella D, Mjøen T, et al. (2013) Development of the Viking Speech Scale to classify the speech of children with cerebral palsy. *Res Dev Disabil,* 34, 3202–10.

65. Virella D, Pennington L, Andersen GL, et al. (2016) Classification systems of communication for use in epidemiological surveillance of children with cerebral palsy. *Dev Med Child Neurol,* 58, 285–91.

66. Sellers D, Mandy A, Pennington L, Hankins M, Morris C (2014) Development and reliability of a system to classify the eating and drinking ability of people with cerebral palsy. *Dev Med Child Neurol,* 56, 245–51.

67. Sellers D, Pennington L, Bryant E, et al. (2022) Mini-EDACS: Development of the Eating and Drinking Ability Classification System for young children with cerebral palsy. *Dev Med Child Neurol,* 64, 897–906.

68. Baranello G, Signorini S, Tinelli F, et al. (2020) Visual Function Classification System for children with cerebral palsy: Development and validation. *Dev Med Child Neurol,* 62, 104–110.

69. Paulson A, Vargus-Adams J (2017) Overview of four functional classification systems commonly used in cerebral palsy. *Children,* 4, 1–10.

70. Piscitelli D, Ferrarello F, Ugolini A, Verola S, Pellicciari L (2021) Measurement properties of the Gross Motor Function Classification System, Gross Motor Function Classification System-expanded & revised, Manual Ability Classification System, and Communication Function Classification System in cerebral palsy: A systematic review with meta-analysis. *Dev Med Child Neurol,* 63, 1251–1261.

71. Shevell M (2019) Cerebral palsy to cerebral palsy spectrum disorder: Time for a name change? *Neurology,* 92, 233–35.

72. Holsbeeke L, Ketelaar M, Schoemaker MM, Gorter JW (2009) Capacity, capability, and performance: Different constructs or three of a kind? *Arch Phys Med Rehabil,* 90, 849–55.

73. Rosenbaum P, Gorter JW (2012) The 'F-words' in childhood disability: I swear this is how we should think! *Child Care Health Dev,* 38, 457–63.

74. Brenner M, Kidston C, Hilliard C, et al. (2018) Children's complex care needs: A systematic concept analysis of multidisciplinary language. *Eur J Pediatr,* 177, 1641–1652.

75. Glader L, Plews-Ogan J, Agrawal R (2016) Children with medical complexity: Creating a framework for care based on the international classification of functioning, disability and health. *Dev Med Child Neurol,* 58, 1116–1123.

76. Nuckolls GH, Kinnett K, Dayanidhi S, et al. (2020) Conference report on contractures in musculoskeletal and neurological conditions. *Muscle Nerve,* 61, 740–744.

77. Howard J, Soo B, Graham HK, et al. (2005) Cerebral palsy in Victoria: Motor types, topography and gross motor function. *J Paediatr Child Health,* 41, 479–83.

78. Carnahan K, Arner M, Hagglund G (2007) Association between gross motor function (GMFCS) and manual ability (MACS) in children with cerebral palsy. A population-based study of 359 children. *BMC Musculoskelet Disord,* 8, 1–7.

79. Rice J, Russo R, Halbert J, Van Essen P, Haan E (2009) Motor function in 5-year-old children with cerebral palsy in the South Australian population. *Dev Med Child Neurol,* 51, 551–6.

80. Delacy MJ, Reid SM, Australian Cerebral Palsy Register Group (2016) Profile of associated impairments at age 5 years in Australia by cerebral palsy subtype and Gross Motor Function Classification System level for birth years 1996 to 2005. *Dev Med Child Neurol,* 58, 50–6.

81. CanChild (2024) *Family-centred service.* [online] Available at: <https://canchild.ca/en/research-in-practice/family-centred-service> [Accessed February 22 2024].

82. Gillette Children's (2018) *Cerebral palsy road map: What to expect as your child grows [pdf].* [online] Available at: <http://gillettechildrens.org/assets/uploads/care-and-conditions/CP_Roadmap.pdf> [Accessed February 22 2024].

83. Sackett DL, Rosenberg WM, Gray JA, Haynes RB, Richardson WS (1996) Evidence based medicine: What it is and what it isn't. *BMJ,* 312, 71–2.

84. Academy of Pediatric Physical Therapy (2019) Fact sheet: The ABCs of pediatric physical therapy. [pdf] Wisconsin, APTA, Available at: <https://pediatricapta.org/includes/fact-sheets/pdfs/FactSheet_ABCsofPediatricPT_2019.pdf?v=2> [Accessed April 24 2024].

85. Agency for Healthcare Research and Quality (2020) The SHARE approach: A model for shared decisionmaking – fact sheet, Available at: <https://www.ahrq.gov/health-literacy/professional-training/shared-decision/tools/factsheet.html> [Accessed February 18 2024].

86. Palisano RJ (2006) A collaborative model of service delivery for children with movement disorders: A framework for evidence-based decision making. *Phys Ther,* 86, 1295–305.

87. Mayston M (2018) More studies are needed in paediatric neurodisability. *Dev Med Child Neurol,* 60, 966.

88. Morris ZS, Wooding S, Grant J (2011) The answer is 17 years, what is the question: Understanding time lags in translational research. *J R Soc Med,* 104, 510–20.

89. Deville C, McEwen I, Arnold SH, Jones M, Zhao YD (2015) Knowledge translation of the Gross Motor Function Classification System among pediatric physical therapists. *Pediatr Phys Ther,* 27, 376–84.

90. Bailes A, Gannotti M, Bellows D, et al. (2018) Caregiver knowledge and preferences for gross motor function information in cerebral palsy. *Dev Med Child Neurol,* 60, 1264–1270.

91. Gross PH, Bailes AF, Horn SD, et al. (2018) Setting a patient-centered research agenda for cerebral palsy: A participatory action research initiative. *Dev Med Child Neurol,* 60, 1278–1284.

92. Wallwiener M, Brucker SY, Wallwiener D, Steering C (2012) Multidisciplinary breast centres in Germany: A review and update of quality assurance through benchmarking and certification. *Arch Gynecol Obstet,* 285, 1671–83.

93. Damiano D, Longo E (2021) Early intervention evidence for infants with or at risk for cerebral palsy: An overview of systematic reviews. *Dev Med Child Neurol,* 63, 771–784.

94. Ogbeiwi O (2018) General concepts of goals and goal-setting in healthcare: A narrative review. *Journal of Management & Organization,* 27, 324–341.

95. Löwing K, Bexelius A, Brogren Carlberg E (2009) Activity focused and goal directed therapy for children with cerebral palsy–do goals make a difference? *Disabil Rehabil,* 31, 1808–16.

96. Phoenix M, Rosenbaum P (2014) Development and implementation of a paediatric rehabilitation care path for hard-to-reach families: A case report. *Child Care Health Dev,* 41, 494–9.

97. Franki I, De Cat J, Deschepper E, et al. (2014) A clinical decision framework for the identification of main problems and treatment goals for ambulant children with bilateral spastic cerebral palsy. *Res Dev Disabil,* 35, 1160–76.

98. Law M, Baptiste S, Carswell A, et al. (2019) *Canadian occupational performance measure.* Ottawa: COMP Inc.

99. Turner-Stokes L (2009) Goal attainment scaling (GAS) in rehabilitation: A practical guide. *Clin Rehabil,* 23, 362–70.

100. Narayanan U, Davidson B, Weir S (2011) The Gait Outcomes Assessment List (GOAL): A new tool to assess cerebral palsy. *Dev Med Child Neurol,* 53, 79.

101. Thomason P, Tan A, Donnan A, et al. (2018) The Gait Outcomes Assessment List (GOAL): Validation of a new assessment of gait function for children with cerebral palsy. *Dev Med Child Neurol,* 60, 618–623.

102. Boyer E, Palmer M, Walt K, Georgiadis A, Stout J (2022) Validation of the Gait Outcomes Assessment List questionnaire and caregiver priorities for individuals with cerebral palsy. *Dev Med Child Neurol,* 64, 379–386.

103. Stout JL, Thill M, Munger ME, Walt K, Boyer ER (2024) Reliability of the Gait Outcomes Assessment List questionnaire. *Dev Med Child Neurol,* 66, 61–69.

104. Narayanan UG, Fehlings D, Weir S, et al. (2006) Initial development and validation of the Caregiver Priorities and Child Health Index of Life with Disabilities (CPCHILD). *Dev Med Child Neurol,* 48, 804–12.

105. Venkateswaran S, Shevell MI (2007) Etiologic profile of spastic quadriplegia in children. *Pediatr Neurol,* 37, 203–8.

106. Gage JR (1991) *Gait analysis in cerebral palsy.* London: Mac Keith Press.

107. Gage JR, Novacheck TF (2001) An update on the treatment of gait problems in cerebral palsy. *J Pediatr Orthop,* 10, 265–74.
108. Keogh J, Sugden DA (1985) *Movement skill development.* London: Macmillan.
109. Day SM, Strauss DJ, Vachon PJ, et al. (2007) Growth patterns in a population of children and adolescents with cerebral palsy. *Dev Med Child Neurol,* 49, 167–71.
110. Brooks J, Day S, Shavelle R, Strauss D (2011) Low weight, morbidity, and mortality in children with cerebral palsy: New clinical growth charts. *Pediatrics,* 128, 299–307.
111. Wright CM, Reynolds L, Ingram E, Cole TJ, Brooks J (2017) Validation of US cerebral palsy growth charts using a UK cohort. *Dev Med Child Neurol,* 59, 933–938.
112. Centers for Disease Control and Prevention (2000a) *2 to 20 years: Girls stature-for-age and weight-for-age percentiles [pdf].* [online] Available at: <https://www.cdc.gov/growthcharts/data/set2clinical/cj41c072.pdf> [Accessed February 22 2024].
113. Centers for Disease Control and Prevention (2009) *Birth to 24 months: Girls length-for-age and weight-for-age percentiles [pdf].* [online] Available at: <https://www.cdc.gov/growthcharts/data/who/GrChrt_Girls_24LW_9210.pdf> [Accessed June 19 2024].
114. Centers for Disease Control and Prevention (2000b) *2 to 20 years: Boys stature-for-age and weight-for-age percentiles [pdf].* [online] Available at: <https://www.cdc.gov/growthcharts/data/set1clinical/cj41l021.pdf> [Accessed February 22 2024].
115. Centers for Disease Control and Prevention (2001) *Birth to 36 months: Boys length-for-age and weight-for-age percentiles [pdf].* [online] Available at: <https://www.cdc.gov/growthcharts/data/set1clinical/cj41l017.pdf> [Accessed February 22 2024].
116. Lance JW (1980) Pathophysiology of spasticity and clinical experience with baclofen. In: Feldman RG, Young RR, Koella WP, editors, *Spasticity: Disordered motor control.* Chicago: Year Book Medical, pp 183–203.
117. Bohannon RW, Smith MB (1987) Interrater reliability of a Modified Ashworth Scale of muscle spasticity. *Phys Ther,* 67, 206–7.
118. Numanoglu A, Gunel MK (2012) Intraobserver reliability of Modified Ashworth Scale and Modified Tardieu Scale in the assessment of spasticity in children with cerebral palsy. *Acta Orthop Traumatol Turc,* 46, 196–200.
119. Gracies JM, Burke K, Clegg NJ, et al. (2010) Reliability of the Tardieu Scale for assessing spasticity in children with cerebral palsy. *Arch Phys Med Rehabil,* 91, 421–8.
120. Barry MJ, VanSwearingen JM, Albright AL (1999) Reliability and responsiveness of the Barry-Albright Dystonia Scale. *Dev Med Child Neurol,* 41, 404–11.
121. Jethwa A, Mink J, Macarthur C, et al. (2010) Development of the Hypertonia Assessment Tool (HAT): A discriminative tool for hypertonia in children. *Dev Med Child Neurol,* 52, 83–7.

122. Knights S, Datoo N, Kawamura A, Switzer L, Fehlings D (2014) Further evaluation of the scoring, reliability, and validity of the Hypertonia Assessment Tool (HAT). *J Child Neurol*, 29, 500–4.

123. Noonan KJ, Farnum CE, Leiferman EM, et al. (2004) Growing pains: Are they due to increased growth during recumbency as documented in a lamb model? *J Pediatr Orthop*, 24, 726–31.

124. Carlon S, Taylor N, Dodd K, Shields N (2013) Differences in habitual physical activity levels of young people with cerebral palsy and their typically developing peers: A systematic review. *Disabil Rehabil*, 35, 647–55.

125. Gough M, Shortland AP (2012) Could muscle deformity in children with spastic cerebral palsy be related to an impairment of muscle growth and altered adaptation? *Dev Med Child Neurol*, 54, 495–9.

126. Nordmark E, Hagglund G, Lauge-Pedersen H, Wagner P, Westbom L (2009) Development of lower limb range of motion from early childhood to adolescence in cerebral palsy: A population-based study. *BMC Med*, 7, 1–11.

127. Smith LR, Chambers HG, Lieber RL (2013) Reduced satellite cell population may lead to contractures in children with cerebral palsy. *Dev Med Child Neurol*, 55, 264–70.

128. Dayanidhi S, Dykstra PB, Lyubasyuk V, et al. (2015) Reduced satellite cell number in situ in muscular contractures from children with cerebral palsy. *J Orthop Res*, 33, 1039–45.

129. Domenighetti AA, Mathewson MA, Pichika R, et al. (2018) Loss of myogenic potential and fusion capacity of muscle stem cells isolated from contractured muscle in children with cerebral palsy. *Am J Physiol Cell Physiol*, 315, 247–257.

130. Barber L, Hastings-Ison T, Baker R, Barrett R, Lichtwark G (2011) Medial gastrocnemius muscle volume and fascicle length in children aged 2 to 5 years with cerebral palsy. *Dev Med Child Neurol*, 53, 543–8.

131. Herskind A, Ritterband-Rosenbaum A, Willerslev-Olsen M, et al. (2016) Muscle growth is reduced in 15-month-old children with cerebral palsy. *Dev Med Child Neurol*, 58, 485–91.

132. Gage JR, Schwartz MH (2009b) Consequences of brain injury on musculoskeletal development. In: Gage JR, Schwartz MH, Koop SE, Novacheck TF, editors, *The identification and treatment of gait problems in cerebral palsy.* London: Mac Keith Press, pp 107–129.

133. Hägglund G, Pettersson K, Czuba T, Persson-Bunke M, Rodby-Bousquet E (2018) Incidence of scoliosis in cerebral palsy. *Acta Orthop*, 89, 443–447.

134. Willoughby KL, Ang SG, Thomason P, et al. (2022) Epidemiology of scoliosis in cerebral palsy: A population-based study at skeletal maturity. *J Paediatr Child Health*, 58, 295–301.

135. Koop SE (2009) Scoliosis in cerebral palsy. *Dev Med Child Neurol*, 51, 92–8.

136. Soo B, Howard JJ, Boyd RN, et al. (2006) Hip displacement in cerebral palsy. *J Bone Joint Surg Am*, 88, 121–9.

137. Graham HK, Thomason P, Novacheck TF (2014) Cerebral palsy. In: Weinstein SL, Flynn JM, editors, *Lovell and Winter's pediatric orthopedics, level 1 and 2.* 7th ed. Philadelphia: Lippincott Williams & Wilkins, pp 484–554.

138. Hägglund G, Alriksson-Schmidt A, Lauge-Pedersen H, et al. (2014) Prevention of dislocation of the hip in children with cerebral palsy: 20-year results of a population-based prevention programme. *Bone Joint J, 96*-B, 1546–52.

139. Hägglund G, Lauge-Pedersen H, Persson Bunke M, Rodby-Bousquet E (2016) Windswept hip deformity in children with cerebral palsy: A population-based prospective follow-up. *J Child Orthop, 10,* 275–9.

140. Karaguzel G, Holick MF (2010) Diagnosis and treatment of osteopenia. *Rev Endocr Metab Disord,* 11, 237–51.

141. Mus-Peters CTR, Huisstede BMA, Noten S, et al. (2018) Low bone mineral density in ambulatory persons with cerebral palsy? A systematic review. *Disabil Rehabil,* 41, 2392–2402.

142. Xie L, Gelfand A, Delclos GL, et al. (2020) Estimated prevalence of asthma in US children with developmental disabilities. *JAMA, 3,* 1–12.

143. Welsh SK, Katwa U (2019) Overview of pulmonary and sleep disorders in children with complex cerebral palsy. In: Glader L, Stevenson R, editors, *Children and youth with complex cerebral palsy: Care and management.* London: Mac Keith Press, pp 155–166.

144. Marpole R, Marie Blackmore A, Gibson N, et al. (2020) Evaluation and management of respiratory illness in children with cerebral palsy. *Front Pediatr,* 8, 333.

145. Gubbay A, Marie Blackmore A (2019) Effects of salivary gland botulinum toxin-A on drooling and respiratory morbidity in children with neurological dysfunction. *Int J Pediatr Otorhinolaryngol,* 124, 124–128.

146. Cross J, Elender F, Barton G, et al. (2012) Evaluation of the effectiveness of manual chest physiotherapy techniques on quality of life at six months post exacerbation of COPD (MATREX): A randomised controlled equivalence trial. *BMC Pulm Med,* 12, 1–9.

147. Saghaleini SH, Dehghan K, Shadvar K, et al. (2018) Pressure ulcer and nutrition. *Indian J Crit Care Med,* 22, 283–289.

148. Bickley M, Delaney E, Intagliata V (2019) Feeding and nutrition. In: Glader L, Stevenson R, editors, *Children and youth with complex cerebral palsy: Care and management.* London: Mac Keith Press, pp 107–207.

149. American Speech-Language-Hearing Association (2024) *Feeding and swallowing disorders in children.* [online] Available at: <https://www.asha.org/public/speech/swallowing/feeding-and-swallowing-disorders-in-children/> [Accessed February 27 2024].

150. Martínez De Zabarte Fernández JM, Ros Arnal I, Peña Segura JL, García Romero R, Rodríguez Martínez G (2020) Nutritional status of a population with moderate-severe cerebral palsy: Beyond the weight. *Anales de Pediatría (English Edition),* 92, 192–199.

151. American College of Gastroenterology (2024) *Percutaneous endoscopic gastrostomy (PEG).* [online] Available at: <https://gi.org/topics/percutaneous-endoscopic-gastrostomy-peg/> [Accessed February 27 2024].

152. Gantasala S, Sullivan PB, Thomas AG (2013) Gastrostomy feeding versus oral feeding alone for children with cerebral palsy. *Cochrane Database Syst Rev,* 1–15.

153. National Institute of Diabetes and Digestive and Kidney Diseases (2020) *Definition and facts for GER and GERD* [online] Available at: <https://www .niddk.nih.gov/health-information/digestive-diseases/acid-reflux-ger-gerd-adults> [Accessed February 27 2024].

154. Gjikopulli A, Kutsch E, Berman L, Prestowitz S (2018) Gastroesophageal reflux in the child with cerebral palsy. In: Miller F, Bachrach S, Lennon N, O'Neil ME, editors, *Cerebral palsy.* Cham: Springer, pp 1–15.

155. Rosen R, Vandenplas Y, Singendonk M, et al. (2018) Pediatric gastroesophageal reflux clinical practice guidelines: Joint recommendations of the North American Society for Pediatric Gastroenterology, Hepatology, and Nutrition and the European Society for Pediatric Gastroenterology, Hepatology, and Nutrition. *J Pediatr Gastroenterol Nutr, 66,* 516–554.

156. National Institute of Diabetes and Digestive and Kidney Diseases (2018) *Definition & facts for constipation.* [online] Available at: <https://www.niddk .nih.gov/health-information/digestive-diseases/constipation/definition-facts> [Accessed February 27 2024].

157. Beinvogl B, Mobassaleh M (2019) Gastrointestinal issues In: Glader L, Stevenson R, editors, *Children and youth with complex cerebral palsy: Care and management.* London: Mac Keith Press, pp 131–152.

158. Svedberg LE, Englund E, Malker H, Stener-Victorin E (2008) Parental perception of cold extremities and other accompanying symptoms in children with cerebral palsy. *Eur J Paediatr Neurol, 12,* 89–96.

159. Elawad MA, Sullivan PB (2001) Management of constipation in children with disabilities. *Dev Med Child Neurol, 43,* 829–32.

160. Eriksson E, Hagglund G, Alriksson-Schmidt AI (2020) Pain in children and adolescents with cerebral palsy–a cross-sectional register study of 3545 individuals. *BMC Neurol, 20,* 1–9.

161. Vinkel MN, Rackauskaite G, Finnerup NB (2022) Classification of pain in children with cerebral palsy. *Dev Med Child Neurol, 64,* 447–452.

162. Wright AJ, Fletcher O, Scrutton D, Baird G (2016) Bladder and bowel continence in bilateral cerebral palsy: A population study. *J Pediatr Urol, 12,* 1–8.

163. Vargus-Adams J (2020) Cerebral palsy. In: Murphy K, Houtrow J, McMahon M, editors, *Pediatric rehabilitation: Principles and practice.* Springer Publishing Company, pp 319–347.

164. Murphy KP, Boutin SA, Ide KR (2012) Cerebral palsy, neurogenic bladder, and outcomes of lifetime care. *Dev Med Child Neurol, 54,* 945–50.

165. Huff JS, Murr N (2023) *Seizure.* [e-book] Treasure Island, StatPearls Publishing. Available at: National Library of Medicine <https://www.ncbi.nlm.nih.gov/ books/NBK430765/> [Accessed February 9 2024].

166. International League Against Epilepsy (2014) *Definition of epilepsy 2014.* [online] Available at: <https://www.ilae.org/guidelines/definition-and-classification/ definition-of-epilepsy-2014> [Accessed March 4 2024].

167. Sellier E, Uldall P, Calado E, et al. (2012) Epilepsy and cerebral palsy: Characteristics and trends in children born in 1976–1998. *Eur J Paediatr Neurol, 16,* 48–55.

168. Pavone P, Gulizia C, Le Pira A, et al. (2020) Cerebral palsy and epilepsy in children: Clinical perspectives on a common comorbidity. *Children*, 8, 1–11.

169. El-Tallawy HN, Farghaly WM, Shehata GA, Badry R, Rageh TA (2014) Epileptic and cognitive changes in children with cerebral palsy: An Egyptian study. *Neuropsychiatr Dis Treat*, 10, 971–5.

170. Mytinger J, Goodkin H (2019) Seizures and epilepsy in children with cerebral palsy. In: Glader L, Stevenson R, editors, *Children and youth with complex cerebral palsy: Care and management.* London: Mac Keith Press, pp 239–248.

171. International League Against Epilepsy (2024) *International league against epilepsy.* [online] Available at: <https://www.ilae.org> [Accessed February 27 2024].

172. Pavlova MK, Ng M, Allen RM, et al. (2021) Proceedings of the sleep and epilepsy workgroup: Section 2 comorbidities: Sleep related comorbidities of epilepsy. *Epilepsy Curr*, 21, 210–214.

173. Giorelli AS, Passos P, Carnaval T, Gomes Mda M (2013) Excessive daytime sleepiness and epilepsy: A systematic review. *Epilepsy Res Treat*, 1–9.

174. Novak I, Hines M, Goldsmith S, Barclay R (2012) Clinical prognostic messages from a systematic review on cerebral palsy. *Pediatrics*, 130, 1285–312.

175. National Institute of Neurological Disorders and Stroke (2023a) *Sleep apnea.* [online] Available at: <https://www.ninds.nih.gov/health-information/disorders/sleep-apnea> [Accessed February 27 2024].

176. Yamaguchi R, Nicholson Perry K, Hines M (2013) Pain, pain anxiety and emotional and behavioural problems in children with cerebral palsy. *Disability Rehabilitation*, 36, 125–30.

177. Hauer J (2019) Pain and irritability. In: Glader L, Stevenson R, editors, *Children and youth with complex cerebral palsy: Care and management.* London: Mac Keith Press, pp 227–237.

178. World Health Organisation (2020) *Palliative care.* [online] Available at: <https://www.who.int/news-room/fact-sheets/detail/palliative-care> [Accessed February 27 2024].

179. Collins M (2014) Strabismus in cerebral palsy: When and why to operate. *Am Orthopt J*, 64, 17–20.

180. Frazier H (2019) Cognitive and sensory impairment. In: Glader L, Stevenson R, editors, *Children and youth with complex cerebral palsy: Care and management.* London: Mac Keith Press, pp 187–193.

181. Rosenbaum P, Rosenbloom L, Mayston M (2012) Therapists and therapies in cerebral palsy. In: Rosenbaum P, Rosenbloom L, editors, *Cerebral palsy: From diagnosis to adulthood.* London: Mac Keith Press, pp 124–148.

182. World Confederation for Physical Therapy (2024) *What is physiotherapy?* [online] Available at: <https://world.physio/resources/what-is-physiotherapy> [Accessed February 22 2024].

183. Fowler EG, Ho TW, Nwigwe AI, Dorey FJ (2001) The effect of quadriceps femoris muscle strengthening exercises on spasticity in children with cerebral palsy. *Phys Ther*, 81, 1215–23.

184. Rosen L, Plummer T, Sabet A, Lange ML, Livingstone R (2023) RESNA position on the application of power mobility devices for pediatric users. *Assistive Technology*, 35, 14–22.

185. Butler C (1986) Effects of powered mobility on self-initiated behaviors of very young children with locomotor disability. *Dev Med Child Neurol*, 28, 325–32.

186. Anderson DI, Campos JJ, Witherington DC, et al. (2013) The role of locomotion in psychological development. *Frontiers in Psychology*, 4, 1–17.

187. Pin T, Dyke P, Chan M (2006) The effectiveness of passive stretching in children with cerebral palsy. *Dev Med Child Neurol*, 48, 855–62.

188. American Occupational Therapy Association (2024) *Patients & clients: Learn about occupational therapy.* [online] Available at: <https://www.aota.org/about/what-is-ot> [Accessed February 22 2024].

189. Bailes A, Reder R, Burch C (2008) Development of guidelines for determining frequency of therapy services in a pediatric medical setting. *Pediatr Phys Ther*, 20, 194–8.

190. Gillette Children's (2024) *Episodes of care in childhood and adolescence.* [online] Available at: <https://www.gillettechildrens.org/assets/REHA-006_EOC_English.pdf> [Accessed January 19 2024].

191. Novak I, McIntyre S, Morgan C, et al. (2013) A systematic review of interventions for children with cerebral palsy: State of the evidence. *Dev Med Child Neurol*, 55, 885–910.

192. Verschuren O, Peterson MD, Balemans AC, Hurvitz EA (2016) Exercise and physical activity recommendations for people with cerebral palsy. *Dev Med Child Neurol*, 58, 798–808.

193. Hulst RY, Gorter JW, Obeid J, et al. (2023) Accelerometer-measured physical activity, sedentary behavior, and sleep in children with cerebral palsy and their adherence to the 24-hour activity guidelines. *Dev Med Child Neurol*, 65, 393–405.

194. Morgan P, Cleary S, Dutia I, Bow K, Shields N (2023) Community-based physical activity interventions for adolescents and adults with complex cerebral palsy: A scoping review. *Dev Med Child Neurol*, 65, 1451–1463.

195. World Health Organization (2024a) *Assistive technology.* [online] Available at: <https://www.who.int/news-room/fact-sheets/detail/assistive-technology> [Accessed February 22 2024].

196. Lunsford C, Greenwood J (2019) Seating, mobility, and equipment needs. In: Glader L, Stevenson R, editors, *Children and youth with complex cerebral palsy: Care and management.* London: Mac Keith Press, pp 65–85.

197. Ward M, Johnson C, Klein J, McGeary FJ, Nolin W PM (2021) Orthotics and assistive devices. In: Murphy KP, McMahon MA, Houtrow AJ, editors, *Pediatric rehabilitation principles and practice.* New York: Springer, pp 196–229.

198. Paleg GS, Smith BA, Glickman LB (2013) Systematic review and evidence-based clinical recommendations for dosing of pediatric supported standing programs. *Pediatr Phys Ther*, 25, 232–47.

199. American Speech-Language-Hearing Association (nd) *Augmentative and alternative communication (AAC).* [online] Available at: <https://www.asha.org/public/speech/disorders/aac/> [Accessed February 27 2024].

200. Owen E, Rahlin M, Kane K (2023) Content validity of a collaborative goal-setting pictorial tool for children who wear ankle-foot orthoses: A modified Delphi consensus study. *JPO Journal of Prosthetics and Orthotics*, 32, 89–98.

201. Ward ME (2009) Pharmacologic treatment with oral medications. In: Gage JR, Schwartz MH, Koop SE, Novacheck TF, editors, *The identification and treatment of gait problems in cerebral palsy*. London: Mac Keith Press, pp 349–362.

202. Molenaers G, Desloovere K (2009) Pharmacologic treatment with botulinum toxin. In: Gage JR, Schwartz MH, Koop SE, Novacheck TF, editors, *The identification and treatment of gait problems in cerebral palsy*. London: Mac Keith Press, pp 363–380.

203. Multani I, Manji J, Hastings-Ison T, Khot A, Graham K (2019) Botulinum toxin in the management of children with cerebral palsy. *Paediatr Drugs*, 21, 261–281.

204. Shore BJ, Thomason P, Reid SM, Shrader MW, Graham HK (2021) Cerebral palsy. In: Weinstein S, Flynn J, Crawford H, editors, *Lovell and Winter's pediatric orthopedics, level 1 and 2*. 8th ed. Philadelphia: Wolters Kluwer, pp 508–589.

205. Love SC, Novak I, Kentish M, et al. (2010) Botulinum toxin assessment, intervention and after-care for lower limb spasticity in children with cerebral palsy: International consensus statement. *Eur J Neurol*, 17, 9–37.

206. Molenaers G, Fagard K, Van Campenhout A, Desloovere K (2013) Botulinum toxin A treatment of the lower extremities in children with cerebral palsy. *J Child Orthop*, 7, 383–7.

207. Fortuna R, Horisberger M, Vaz MA, Herzog W (2013) Do skeletal muscle properties recover following repeat onabotulinum toxin A injections? *J Biomech*, 46, 2426–33.

208. Fortuna R, Vaz MA, Sawatsky A, Hart DA, Herzog W (2015) A clinically relevant BTX-A injection protocol leads to persistent weakness, contractile material loss, and an altered mRNA expression phenotype in rabbit quadriceps muscles. *J Biomech*, 48, 1700–6.

209. Mathevon L, Michel F, Decavel P, et al. (2015) Muscle structure and stiffness assessment after botulinum toxin type A injection. A systematic review. *Ann Phys Rehabil Med*, 58, 343–50.

210. Valentine J, Stannage K, Fabian V, et al. (2016) Muscle histopathology in children with spastic cerebral palsy receiving botulinum toxin type A. *Muscle Nerve*, 53, 407–14.

211. Alexander C, Elliott C, Valentine J, et al. (2018) Muscle volume alterations after first botulinum neurotoxin A treatment in children with cerebral palsy: A 6-month prospective cohort study. *Dev Med Child Neurol*, 60, 1165–1171.

212. Schless SH, Cenni F, Bar-On L, et al. (2019) Medial gastrocnemius volume and echo-intensity after botulinum neurotoxin A interventions in children with spastic cerebral palsy. *Dev Med Child Neurol*, 61, 783–790.

213. Tang MJ, Graham HK, Davidson KE (2021) Botulinum toxin A and osteosarcopenia in experimental animals: A scoping review. *Toxins*, 13, 1–13.

214. Gillette Children's (2013) *Pediatric spasticity management*. St. Paul: Gillette Children's Hospital. Unpublished.

215. Gormley M, S D (2021) Hypertonia. In: Murphy KP, McMahon MA, Houtrow AJ, editors, *Pediatric rehabilitation: Principles and practices*. New York: Springer, pp 100–124.

216. Abdel Ghany W, Nada M, Mahran M, et al. (2016) Combined anterior and posterior lumbar rhizotomy for treatment of mixed dystonia and spasticity in children with cerebral palsy. *Neurosurgery, 79,* 336–44.

217. Gillette Children's (2023b) *Deep brain stimulation (DBS) for children.* [online] Available at: <https://www.gillettechildrens.org/conditions-care/deep-brain -stimulation-dbs> [Accessed February 27 2024].

218. Fehlings D, Brown L, Harvey A, et al. (2018) Pharmacological and neurosurgical interventions for managing dystonia in cerebral palsy: A systematic review. *Dev Med Child Neurol, 60,* 356–366.

219. Jung NH, Pereira B, Nehring I, et al. (2014) Does hip displacement influence health-related quality of life in children with cerebral palsy? *Dev Neurorehabil, 17,* 420–5.

220. American Academy for Cerebral Palsy and Developmental Medicine (2017) *Hip surveillance in cerebral palsy.* [online] Available at: <https://www.aacpdm .org/publications/care-pathways/hip-surveillance-in-cerebral-palsy> [Accessed February 22 2024].

221. Hägglund G, Andersson S, Düppe H, et al. (2005) Prevention of dislocation of the hip in children with cerebral palsy. The first ten years of a population-based prevention programme. *J Bone Joint Surg Br, 87,* 95–101.

222. Mergler S (2018) Bone status in cerebral palsy. In: Panteliadis CP, editor, *Cerebral palsy: A multidisciplinary approach.* Cham: Springer International Publishing, pp 253–257.

223. McCarthy JJ, D'Andrea LP, Betz RR, Clements DH (2006) Scoliosis in the child with cerebral palsy. *J Am Acad Orthop Surg, 14,* 367–75.

224. Koop SE (2009) Musculoskeletal growth and development. In: Gage JR, Schwartz MH, Koop SE, Novacheck TF, editors, *The identification and treatment of gait problems in cerebral palsy.* London: Mac Keith Press, pp 21–30.

225. Miyanji F, Nasto LA, Sponseller PD, et al. (2018) Assessing the risk-benefit ratio of scoliosis surgery in cerebral palsy: Surgery is worth it. *JBJS, 100,* 556–563.

226. Miller DJ, Flynn JJM, Pasha S, et al. (2020) Improving health-related quality of life for patients with nonambulatory cerebral palsy: Who stands to gain from scoliosis surgery? *J Pediatr Orthop, 40,* 186–192.

227. Jain A, Sullivan BT, Shah SA, et al. (2018) Caregiver perceptions and health-related quality-of-life changes in cerebral palsy patients after spinal arthrodesis. *Spine, 43,* 1052–1056.

228. American Psychiatric Association (2024) *What is intellectual disability.* [online] Available at: <https://www.psychiatry.org/patients-families/intellectual-disability> [Accessed July 27 2024].

229. Saad M (2019) Defining and determining intellectual disability insights from DSM-5. *International Journal of Psycho-Educational Sciences, 8,* 51–54.

230. Semrud-Clikeman M, Teeter Ellison PA (2009) *Child Neuropsychology.* New York: Springer.

231. World Health Organization (2022) *Mental health.* [online] Available at: <https:// www.who.int/news-room/fact-sheets/detail/mental-health-strengthening-our -response> [Accessed February 22 2024].

232. Bjorgaas H, Hysing M, Elgen I (2012) Psychiatric disorders among children with cerebral palsy at school starting age. *Res Dev Disabil,* 33, 1287–93.

233. Downs J, Blackmore A, Epstein A, et al. (2017) The prevalence of mental health disorders and symptoms in children and adolescents with cerebral palsy: A systematic review and meta-analysis. *Dev Med Child Neurol,* 60, 30–38.

234. Rackauskaite G, Bilenberg N, Uldall P, Bech BH, Ostergaard J (2020) Prevalence of mental disorders in children and adolescents with cerebral palsy: Danish nationwide follow-up study. *Eur J Paediatr Neurol,* 27, 98–103.

235. Centers for Disease Control and Prevention (2022) *Prevalence of cerebral palsy, co-occurring autism spectrum disorders, and motor functioning.* [online] Available at: <https://www.cdc.gov/ncbddd/cp/features/prevalence.html> [Accessed January 19 2024].

236. Bahl A, Freeman K (2019) Challenging behaviors, sleep and toileting. In: Glader L, Stevenson R, editors, *Children and youth with complex cerebral palsy: Care and management.* London: Mac Keith Press, pp 195–208.

237. Noritz G, Davidson L, Steingass K, The Council on Children with Disabilities, The American Academy for Cerebral Palsy and Developmental Medicine (2022) Providing a primary care medical home for children and youth with cerebral palsy. *American Academy of Pediatrics,* 150, 1–54.

238. Worley G, Houlihan CM, Herman-Giddens ME, et al. (2002) Secondary sexual characteristics in children with cerebral palsy and moderate to severe motor impairment: A cross-sectional survey. *Pediatrics,* 110, 897–902.

239. Gray S (2019) Adolescence and sexuality. In: Glader L, Stevenson R, editors, *Children and youth with complex cerebral palsy: Care and management.* London: Mac Keith Press, pp 263–273.

240. Flavin M, Shore BJ, Miller P, Gray S (2019) Hormonal contraceptive prescription in young women with cerebral palsy. *J Adolesc Health,* 65, 405–409.

241. Christian CA, Reddy DS, Maguire J, Forcelli PA (2020) Sex differences in the epilepsies and associated comorbidities: Implications for use and development of pharmacotherapies. *Pharmacol Rev,* 72, 767–800.

242. Manski R, Dennis A (2014) A mixed-methods exploration of the contraceptive experiences of female teens with epilepsy. *Seizure,* 23, 629–35.

243. Majnemer A, Shikako-Thomas K, Shevell MI, et al. (2013) Pursuit of complementary and alternative medicine treatments in adolescents with cerebral palsy. *J Child Neurol,* 28, 1443–1447.

244. Graham HK (2014) Cerebral palsy prevention and cure: Vision or mirage? A personal view. *J Paediatr Child Health,* 50, 89–90.

245. Wehmeyer ML, Palmer S (2003) Adult outcomes for students with cognitive disabilities three-years after high school: The impact of self-determination. *Education and Training in Developmental Disabilities,* 38, 131–144.

246. Brooks JC, Strauss DJ, Shavelle RM, et al. (2014) Recent trends in cerebral palsy survival. Part II: Individual survival prognosis. *Dev Med Child Neurol,* 56, 1065–71.

247. Rosenthal M (2022) Life expectancy and its adjustment in cerebral palsy with severe impairment: Are we doing this right? *Dev Med Child Neurol,* 64, 709–714.

248. World Health Organization (2024b) *Adolescent health.* [online] Available at: <https://www.who.int/health-topics/adolescent-health#tab=tab_1> [Accessed February 22 2024].

249. Liptak GS (2008) Health and well being of adults with cerebral palsy. *Curr Opin Neurol,* 21, 136–42.

250. Centers for Disease Control and Prevention (2020) *Disability and health related conditions.* [online] Available at: <https://www.cdc.gov/ncbddd/disabilityand health/relatedconditions.html> [Accessed January 19 2024].

251. Wu YW, Mehravari AS, Numis AL, Gross P (2015) Cerebral palsy research funding from the National Institutes of Health, 2001 to 2013. *Dev Med Child Neurol,* 57, 936–41.

252. Tosi LL, Maher N, Moore DW, Goldstein M, Aisen ML (2009) Adults with cerebral palsy: A workshop to define the challenges of treating and preventing secondary musculoskeletal and neuromuscular complications in this rapidly growing population. *Dev Med Child Neurol,* 51, 2–11.

253. Santilli V, Bernetti A, Mangone M, Paoloni M (2014) Clinical definition of sarcopenia. *Clin Cases Miner Bone Metab,* 11, 177–80.

254. Ni Lochlainn M, Bowyer RCE, Steves CJ (2018) Dietary protein and muscle in aging people: The potential role of the gut microbiome. *Nutrients,* 10, 929.

255. World Health Organization (2023) *Noncommunicable diseases.* [online] Available at: <https://www.who.int/news-room/fact-sheets/detail/ noncommunicable-diseases> [Accessed February 22 2024].

256. Sheridan KJ (2009) Osteoporosis in adults with cerebral palsy. *Dev Med Child Neurol,* 51 Suppl 4, 38–51.

257. Ryan JM, Albairami F, Hamilton T, et al. (2023) Prevalence and incidence of chronic conditions among adults with cerebral palsy: A systematic review and meta-analysis. *Dev Med Child Neurol,* 65, 1174–1189.

258. Peterson MD, Ryan JM, Hurvitz EA, Mahmoudi E (2015) Chronic conditions in adults with cerebral palsy. *Jama,* 314, 2303–5.

259. Jonsson U, Eek MN, Sunnerhagen KS, Himmelmann K (2021) Health conditions in adults with cerebral palsy: The association with CP subtype and severity of impairments. *Frontiers in Neurology,* 12, 1–10.

260. Smith KJ, Peterson MD, O'Connell NE, et al. (2019) Risk of depression and anxiety in adults with cerebral palsy. *JAMA Neurol,* 76, 294–300.

261. Cremer N, Hurvitz E, Peterson M (2017) Multimorbidity in middle-aged adults with cerebral palsy. *Am J Med,* 130, 9–15.

262. Jahnsen R, Villien L, Aamodt G, Stanghelle J, Inger H (2003) Physiotherapy and physical activity–experiences of adults with cerebral palsy, with implications for children. *Advances in Physiotherapy,* 5, 21–32.

263. Hilberink SR, Roebroeck ME, Nieuwstraten W, et al. (2007) Health issues in young adults with cerebral palsy: Towards a life-span perspective. *J Rehabil Med,* 39, 605–11.

264. Ryan JM, Crowley VE, Hensey O, McGahey A, Gormley J (2014) Waist circum-ference provides an indication of numerous cardiometabolic risk factors in adults with cerebral palsy. *Arch Phys Med Rehabil,* 95, 1540–6.

265. Putz C, Döderlein L, Mertens EM, et al. (2016) Multilevel surgery in adults with cerebral palsy. *Bone Joint J,* 98b, 282–8.

266. Cassidy C, Campbell N, Madady M, Payne M (2016) Bridging the gap: The role of physiatrists in caring for adults with cerebral palsy. *Disabil Rehabil,* 38, 493–8.

267. Pettersson K, Rodby-Bousquet E (2021) Living conditions and social outcomes in adults with cerebral palsy. *Front Neurol,* 12, 1–12.

268. Murphy KP (2018) Comment on: Cerebral palsy, non-communicable diseases, and lifespan care. *Dev Med Child Neurol,* 60, 733.

269. Rosenbaum P (2019) Diagnosis in developmental disability: A perennial challenge, and a proposed middle ground. *Dev Med Child Neurol,* 61, 620.

270. Schuh L (2023) *Personal communication.*

271. Imms C, Dodd KJ (2010) What is cerebral palsy? In: Dodd KJ, Imms C, Taylor NF, editors, *Physiotherapy and occupational therapy for people with cerebral palsy: A problem-based approach to assessment and management.* London: Mac Keith Press, pp 7–30.

272. Ryan JM, Allen E, Gormley J, Hurvitz EA, Peterson MD (2018) The risk, burden, and management of non-communicable diseases in cerebral palsy: A scoping review. *Dev Med Child Neurol,* 60, 753–764.

Index

Abbreviations used in index: CP cerebral palsy; ICF International Classification of Functioning, Disability and Health; ROM range of motion. Figures and tables indicated by page numbers in italics.